ORTHOTICS IN FUNCTIONAL REHABILITATION OF THE LOWER LIMB

ORTHOTICS IN FUNCTIONAL REHABILITATION OF THE LOWER LIMB

DEBORAH A. NAWOCZENSKI, PhD, PT
Associate Professor
Department of Physical Therapy
Ithaca College–University of Rochester Campus
Rochester, New York

MARCIA E. EPLER, PhD, PT, ATC
Assistant Professor
Department of Physical Therapy
Philadelphia College of Pharmacy and Science
Philadelphia, Pennsylvania

SAUNDERS
An Imprint of Elsevier

SAUNDERS
An Imprint of Elsevier
The Curtis Center
Independence Square West
Philadelphia, PA 19106

Library of Congress Cataloging-in-Publication Data

Orthotics in functional rehabilitation of the lower limb / [edited by] Deborah
Nawoczenski, Marcia Epler.

p.   cm.

Includes index.

ISBN 0–7216–6134–3

1. Leg—Mechanical properties.   2. Orthopedic apparatus.   3. Physically
   handicapped—Rehabilitation.   I. Nawoczenski, Deborah A.   II. Epler,
   Marcia E.

[DNLM: 1. Leg Injuries—rehabilitation.   2. Orthotic Devices.   WE 850 077
1997]

RD779.078   1997   617.3′9803—dc20

DNLM/DLC   96–25618

ORTHOTICS IN FUNCTIONAL REHABILITATION
OF THE LOWER LIMB   ISBN 0–7216–6134–3

Printed in the United States of America.

Last digit is the print number: 9   8   7   6   5

Dedicated to our cherished mentors
Walt and Mary
Betty and Bill

TJ ANTICH, MS, PT
Clinical Director/Principal, Newtown Square Sports Physical Therapy
Newton Square, Pennsylvania
MacDade Orthopaedic & Sports Physical Therapy
Milmont Park, Pennsylvania
Orthoses for the Knee: The Tibiofemoral Joint

BARBARA C. BELYEA, MS, PT
Clinical Assistant Professor
Department of Physical Therapy
Ithaca College
Ithaca, New York
Orthoses for the Knee: The Patellofemoral Joint

MARCIA E. EPLER, PhD, PT, ATC
Assistant Professor
Department of Physical Therapy
Philadelphia College of Pharmacy and Science
Philadelphia, Pennsylvania
Orthoses for the Ankle

KATHRYN P. HEMSLEY, PT, ATC, OCS
Adjunct Faculty, Beaver College
Physical Therapy Program
Glenside, Pennsylvania
Senior Staff Therapist/Athletic Trainer
Temple University Department of Orthopaedics
Philadelphia, Pennsylvania
Physical Therapist
Bryn Mawr Rehab, Malvern, Pennsylvania
Protective Padding and Adhesive Strapping

PETER J. MILLER, MHS, PT
Assistant Professor
Department of Physical Therapy
Philadelphia College of Pharmacy and Science
Philadelphia, Pennsylvania
Orthoses for the Pelvic and Hip Region

DEBORAH A. NAWOCZENSKI, PhD, PT
Associate Professor
Department of Physical Therapy
Ithaca College–University of Rochester Campus
Rochester, New York
Introduction to Orthotics: Rationale for Treatment; Orthoses for the Foot

MEG STANGER, MS, PT, PCS
Assistant Professor
Department of Physical Therapy
Philadelphia College of Pharmacy and Science
Philadelphia, Pennsylvania
Use of Orthoses in Pediatrics

CYNTHIA M. ZABLOTNY, MS, PT, NCS
Adjunct Assistant Professor
Department of Physical Therapy
Ithaca College–University of Rochester Campus
Rochester, New York
Staff Physical Therapist
Brain Injury Rehabilitation Program
St. Mary's Hospital
Rochester, New York
Use of Orthoses for the Adult with Neurologic Involvement

This text is designed to be a comprehensive clinical resource for the health-care provider involved in the orthotic prescription process for lower-limb dysfunction. Orthotic intervention strategies are featured for both adult and pediatric populations having orthopedic and/or neurologic impairment. Our primary objective is to present information about orthotic appliances that is based on empirical data and evidence of their effectiveness in clinical trials. This information will guide practitioners treating patients with musculoskeletal and neurologic disorders.

An introductory chapter provides an overview of orthotic principles and characteristics of materials frequently used in orthotic fabrication. A regional approach to orthotic management focusing on musculoskeletal disorders of the hip, knee (patellofemoral and tibiofemoral joints), ankle, and foot is presented in subsequent chapters. In cases in which permanent or definitive orthoses may not be warranted, or for prophylactic indications, adhesive strapping techniques offer an alternative to traditional orthotic management of musculoskeletal injuries. These adhesive strapping techniques are presented in an extensively illustrated chapter that follows regional orthotic management. The primary focus of the final two chapters of the text is on orthotic considerations for adult and pediatric patients with neurologic dysfunction. Critical attention is given to the impact of orthoses on mobility and function during gait.

Each chapter contains illustrations of the orthoses appropriate to the selected anatomic region. This feature is beneficial for the clinician or student who may have little experience with the orthotic devices. When appropriate, tables are included to highlight key features of the orthoses and present a "quick reference" for the user. The illustrative techniques for lower-limb adhesive strapping provide the clinician with options for rendering support, stabilization, and protection for musculoskeletal injuries in lieu of permanent devices. These strapping techniques may also prove helpful to the clinician who wishes to assess the potential benefit of an orthosis prior to recommendation of a more definitive appliance, should it be necessary.

The book is intended for practitioners across a variety of disciplines involved in the orthotic recommendation process. The content should be appropriate for the student as well as the experienced clinician involved in orthopedics, sports medicine, athletic training, pediatrics, and adult neurologic rehabilitation.

As the text evolved, it became apparent that there are gaps in our understanding of why orthoses are effective. The majority of controlled studies have been directed to the impact of various knee and ankle orthoses on functional performance, primarily in the adult athlete. We hope the material presented in this book not only assists the practitioner in making appropriate choices but also encourages further study of orthotic effectiveness that supports or refutes the use of these devices in patient care.

DEBORAH A. NAWOCZENSKI
MARCIA E. EPLER

Acknowledgments

This text would not have been possible without the support and diligent efforts of our colleagues, friends, and families. We thank our photographers, Barbara Proud, Stan and Sue Wallace, and Kathryn Hemsley, for capturing the images necessary to convey the information provided within the chapters. Thanks also to our illustrator, Larry Ward, who provided the images unable to be captured by the camera. Jim Johnson from Aircast, Inc. has been invaluable in his continued assistance with our projects. We express our appreciation to Mandy Fingerlin, Martha Griswold, Joe Pistorius, and Eileen Dougherty for their assistance in the production of Chapter 7, Protective Padding and Adhesive Strapping, and to Frank Gramaglia of Greiner and Saur, Inc. for his assistance and provision of many of the knee orthoses. Thanks also to Kevin Coloton, Beth Gallagher, John Stemm, and Julie Wallace, who served as models for many of the orthoses pictured in the text. Finally, we thank the authors, who shared their precious time and talent with their contributions to this work.

Contents

ORTHOTICS IN FUNCTIONAL REHABILITATION OF THE LOWER LIMB

CHAPTER 1

Introduction to Orthotics: Rationale for Treatment

DEBORAH A. NAWOCZENSKI

Before prescribing an orthotic appliance, the health care provider should consider the goals of the orthosis, the degrees-of-freedom to be altered or affected, and the forces required to achieve the desired outcomes. Orthotic prescription and fabrication should suggest a dynamic process such that the goals and, therefore, the orthoses reflect the patient's changing needs and functional status.

This chapter addresses the basic principles and rationale for orthotic designs and supportive strapping techniques that are presented in subsequent chapters. A description of orthotic materials is presented, together with a brief overview of the physiologic and financial considerations significant to effective orthotic prescription.

FUNCTIONAL CONSIDERATIONS FOR ORTHOTIC PRESCRIPTION

Goals

When an orthosis is prescribed, the goals may include one or any combination of the following: rest, immobilization, joint protection, control, assisting movement, providing feedback, and correction. These goals are achieved through selected application of forces. If the desired goal is to rest a part of the body, the orthosis must be able to substitute for, or assist with, the action of the muscles. Alternatively, orthotic intervention may be indicated for the purpose of immobilization to reduce pain or provide joint protection immediately following surgery or injury. In these cases, the orthosis substitutes for the lack of intrinsic stability normally achieved by the bony, ligamentous, or muscular components.

The orthotic prescription should take into account whether the purpose of the appliance is to control or to assist movement. A basic understanding of the injured anatomic structures that render certain movements or movement directions unstable is necessary in order to incorporate the appropriate support and rigidity into the orthosis. Consider the person who has weakness of the gastrocnemius-soleus muscle group. The purpose of an ankle-foot orthosis (AFO) in this case may be to control forward tibial motion and to minimize knee instability during the stance phase of gait. Both the height of the AFO and its rigidity are important design considerations in this prescription. Conversely, these same design characteristics may not be appropriate for a person presenting with pretibial muscle weakness. In this case, the primary goal of the AFO is to support the weight of the foot and shoe and to assist toe clearance during the swing phase of gait. The increased height and rigidity of the appliance are less critical in this orthotic prescription because the movement requirements are different.

Orthoses have also been prescribed for the purpose of providing feedback to the user. The potential to increase the afferent input from cutaneous receptors, which in turn may lead to improved position sense, has been considered in both prophylactic and rehabilitative applications.[6] The primary prophylactic use of orthoses has been directed to knee and ankle injury prevention. The findings of investigations assessing prophylactic benefits of knee and ankle orthoses have been mixed[8, 13, 20, 22, 24] and are discussed in Chapters 4 and 5, respectively. Finally, an orthosis may provide correction, utilizing the viscoelastic characteristics of the intervening soft tissues to cause a deformation in bony structures over time.[27]

Degrees-of-Freedom

Before selecting an orthotic device, the health care provider should consider the kinematic characteristics of the region of interest including an analysis of the degrees-of-freedom. This rationale entails an evaluation of the translation along, and rotation about, each of the coordinate axes of the respective segments or joints to be braced. Although most treatment strategies typically address one or two of the six potential degrees-of-freedom, an awareness of all inherent motions and coupled relationships between segments is important in maximizing the effectiveness of the orthosis. Foot orthoses provide a relevant example of attempting to control motion of the foot in the frontal plane and altering motion in another plane. This control is achieved by "posting," or adding a wedge to the orthotic. In view of the coupled rotation between the foot and lower extremity, frontal plane posting techniques have been shown to modify transverse plane rotations of the tibia in patients with certain foot structures.[14]

The attempt to control or to limit two or more degrees-of-freedom continues to present challenges to orthotic designers. Knee orthoses for anterior cruciate injury or repair perhaps represent the best examples of the continual evolution of orthoses in the quest for the optimal appliance that controls both translation and rotation without sacrificing functional performance. These devices are discussed in Chapter 4.

ACHIEVING DESIRED OUTCOMES THROUGH FORCE APPLICATION

The desired outcomes of orthotic intervention are achieved through selected application and transmission of forces via the orthotic appliance. Indirect transmission of force through structures such as muscles, fascia, tendons, fat, viscera, and bone, as well as through footwear, help achieve these outcomes. One important concept underlying many of the strategies in force application is the phenomenon known as creep. Creep is the deformation that follows the initial loading of a viscoelastic material, and it occurs over a period ranging from several seconds to several days.[27] After this period, biologically mediated changes in the mechanical properties of the tissues occur.[27]

With few exceptions, the application of forces to achieve a desired outcome must account for increased pressure at the points of force application. Pressure, which is defined as the total force per unit area, causes greater concern for persons who have sensory or cognitive loss. In general, to avoid pain (given intact sensation) and skin breakdown, forces should be sustained over as large an area of body surface as possible without compromising the goals of the orthosis or the function of the user.

Principles of Force Transmission

The potential for achieving optimal control, correction, stabilization, or assistance via orthotic intervention is accomplished through various design principles. Much of the force transmission is mediated through balanced horizontal or parallel forces, frequently using a three-point loading system.[21] Examples of common three-point loading systems used in orthotic therapies are shown in Figure 1–1. The three forces in this system are applied to a

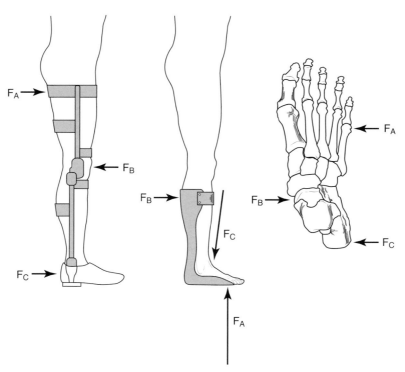

FIGURE 1–1. Examples of three-point force applications. The maximum bending moment occurs at the location of the middle force (F_B) in each example. The forces can be applied through the orthosis, the shoe, or orthosis/shoe combination.

segment, or segments, such that the two forces in one direction (F_A and F_C) are countered by a third opposing force (F_B) located between the other two forces. Because the system is in equilibrium, the sum of the forces and the sum of the bending moments created must be equal to zero. Therefore, the location of force application and the resultant magnitudes are interrelated.

Consider the three forces F_A, F_B, and F_C that may be applied in an orthosis to control excessive genu recurvatum (Fig. 1–2). The magnitudes of the forces at points F_A and F_C are in inverse proportion to their perpendicular distances (D_1 and D_2) from point F_B. In addition, the sum of the forces at points A and C must be equal to the force at point B. If the two anterior pads in a knee-ankle-foot orthosis (KAFO) are placed equidistant from the posterior pad, the force at the posterior pad is twice that of each anterior pad.

This information holds particular clinical relevance to skin pressures and breakdown. To account for differences in force magnitudes, the pad must be proportioned to minimize localized areas of high skin pressures. In the previous example in Figure 1–2, the posterior pad imparts twice the force of the equidistant anterior pads, and it should have greater pad surface area in order to sustain similar skin pressures.

Characteristic features of this three-point system are the bending moment and transverse shear forces created by the applied forces.[3, 4, 21, 27] These loads are created when forces applied to a "rigid" structure are not collinear with

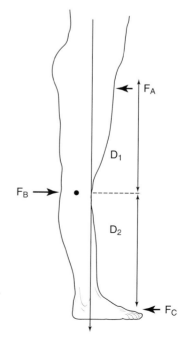

FIGURE 1–2. A three-point loading system for controlling genu recurvatum. The magnitude of force A (F_A) and of force C (F_C) are in inverse proportion to their perpendicular distances (D_1 and D_2) from force B (F_B).

the reacting force. Both the bending moments and the transverse shear forces are important to the design and intended purpose of the orthosis.

The bending moment varies along the length of the structure, being zero under the end forces and greatest under the middle force. This moment can be graphically represented by the triangular bending moment diagram shown in Figure 1–3. The maximum corrective or control potential is applied at the apex of the diagram.[4, 27] Because the bending moment is proportional to the length of the moment arm, the effectiveness of a three-point orthosis is strongly influenced by the location of forces relative to the joint axis. The farther the end forces are from the joint, the greater their moment arms, and the smaller the magnitudes required to produce a given torque at the joint. If the middle force is moved away from the joint center toward one end of the limb, reaction forces of different magnitudes are required to maintain equilibrium. These changes in the location of the maximum bending moment and thus in the effective torque are demonstrated in Figure 1–4.

These same figures also illustrate the transverse shear forces that displace one segment relative to another along the plane of action of the forces. The location and magnitude of the shear forces depend on the external support

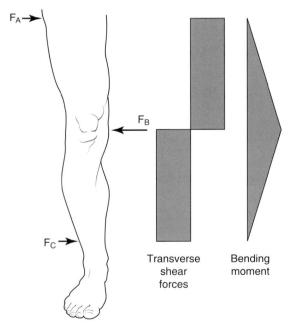

Transverse shear forces

Bending moment

FIGURE 1–3. A three-point loading system with transverse shear forces and bending moment diagrams. The bending moment varies along the length of the structure, being zero under the end forces (F_A and F_C) and maximum under the middle force (F_B). The maximum corrective or control potential is located at the apex of the bending moment diagram. In this figure, the maximum bending moment is located at the medial knee joint, or F_B.

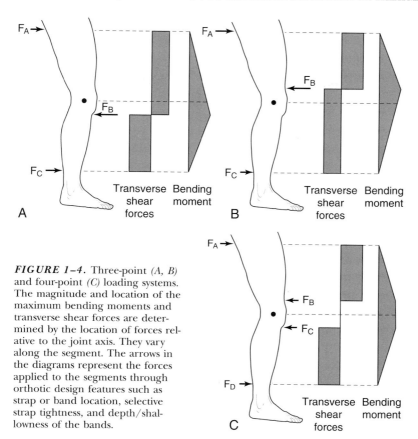

FIGURE 1–4. Three-point *(A, B)* and four-point *(C)* loading systems. The magnitude and location of the maximum bending moments and transverse shear forces are determined by the location of forces relative to the joint axis. They vary along the segment. The arrows in the diagrams represent the forces applied to the segments through orthotic design features such as strap or band location, selective strap tightness, and depth/shallowness of the bands.

reactions generated by the brace and mechanisms of loading.[21] The forces are controlled through orthotic design features such as strap location, selective strap tightness, and depth/shallowness of the bands. In order to minimize shear force at any one point along a segment, the sum of the forces on opposite sides of the segment must be equal to zero.

For other types of loading systems, the bending moment diagram takes on a different shape. In the four-point system shown in Figure 1–4*C*, for example, two horizontal or parallel forces (F_A, F_D) are applied on one side of the segment, and two forces (F_B, F_C) are applied on the other side. In the simplest of cases in which the forces are equal and arranged symmetrically, the structure between the inner pairs of forces (F_B, F_C) is subjected to a constant bending moment.[27] This bending moment diagram can be contrasted with examples of the three-point system in Figure 1–4*A,B*, which demonstrate a varying bending moment having a peak immediately under the middle force.

Principles of Compression and Distraction

Orthotic designs also incorporate other mechanical principles to achieve the desired outcomes. An orthosis may externally support a compressive load or "splint" a structure via soft tissue or fluid compression. The use of an infrapatellar strap for patellar tendinitis (see Chap. 3) and an Achilles tendon strap for Achilles tendinitis (see Chap. 5) are two examples that incorporate the concept of soft tissue compression. Although not clearly understood, the mechanisms by which these straps are effective in pain relief may be due partly to the compression of the tendon. This compression may unload the underlying soft tissues, thereby reducing the tensile stresses on the tendon.[15, 16, 23]

Immobilization and stability may be accomplished through orthotic appliances that provide distraction to the segment. The tension generated as a result of distraction of the ends of a structure increases the lateral stability of the structure. This stability is further enhanced by the application of transverse, or horizontal, forces. Studies of loading behavior on spinal deformities have shown that axial loading by means of distraction, in combination with horizontal force application, provides the most effective correction for deformities associated with scoliosis.[19] This design concept is incorporated into many of the knee orthoses highlighted in Chapter 4. The orthotic device has both proximal and distal fixation points and intervening lateral uprights that provide a point of attachment for various accessory straps. These features offer both immobilization and stability to the joint.

MATERIALS IN ORTHOTIC PRESCRIPTION AND FABRICATION

The ability to successfully manage structural or functional deficits of the lower extremity is enhanced by an understanding of the properties and performance characteristics of different orthotic materials.[9] A review of the literature reveals various descriptions and performance behaviors of materials.[2, 7, 10–12, 17] Materials may be described as soft or flexible, semirigid/semiflexible, or rigid; or they may be described as low-, medium-, or high-density. Materials may also be characterized according to the intended purpose such as corrective, functional, or accommodative. These descriptions provide some information about the structural and performance characteristics of the components used in the orthoses.

Performance characteristics of materials are determined from physical tests of their mechanical behavior. These tests, which provide an indirect gauge of material density, include measurements of compressibility, resiliency, shock absorbency, and energy return. Compressibility is the force required to develop a degree of compression, or the normal force that tends to push a material's fibers together.[5, 10, 27] Resiliency is the ability to "bounce back" after removal of a load, or the restoration of a material's thickness to its original value.[5, 10] The shock-absorbing properties of materials refer to their ability to provide "damping" to an impact load[17] as measured by changes in impact accelerations and ground reaction forces.[12] The energy-return ability can be defined as the percentage of impact energy that is not dissipated by the material, but that provides some "bounce-back" to the user.[12]

The mechanisms of loading behavior used to test materials' characteristics vary across experimental designs and may result in different outcomes of materials' effectiveness. Regardless of the results, careful selection of components for different diagnoses, body weights, and activity levels yields a diverse assortment of finished orthoses to meet different needs of the user. Table 1–1 provides an overview of the characteristics of common materials used in orthotic designs.[5] These materials are described in terms of their density, energy-storing capabilities, and average life span.

Much of the information available on the properties of materials stems from the widespread use of cellular foams and viscoelastic polymers in current foot orthotic therapies. Determining effective management strategies for the insensitive foot has prompted research investigations of the structural and compression properties of the materials in load-bearing applications.[2, 10, 11] The cellular polyethylene foams such as Plastazote (Apex Foot Products, South Hackensack, NJ), Pelite (Active International, Hillside, NJ), Spenco (Spenco Medical Corp., Waco, TX) and Aliplast (Alimed, Dedham, MA) are some of the most common soft materials currently in use. They are generally moldable with the application of heat (varying between 200 and 300°F [93 to 149°C]) and are available in various densities. Their function is usually accommodative because no attempt is made to alter motion through use of these materials. These materials, however, decrease in thickness or

TABLE 1–1
Characteristics of Materials

Material	Density	Energy-Storage Capability	Life Span
PPT	M	M	4–6 months
Spenco	L	L	4–6 months
Plastazote	L	L	4–6 weeks
Aliplast/Plastazote	L/M	L	4–6 months
Cork/leather	H	L	9–12 months
Cork/Spenco	L/H	L	9–12 months
Cork/PPT	M/H	L/M	9–12 months
Cork/Sorbothane	M/H	L/M	9–12 months
Polypropylene	H	H	1–3 years
Rohadur (Polydor)	H	H	1–3 years
Stainless steel	H	M/H	Indefinite

L = low; M = medium; H = high.

"bottom out" fairly rapidly in clinical trials, particularly when used as foot/ shoe interface insoles.[2, 10, 11, 17] The loss of thickness of the moldable polyethylene foam is inversely related to the density of the polyethylene foam.[2, 10, 11] The use of thicker insole interface materials for heavier patients may improve pressure distribution in accommodative insoles, as well as prolong the average life span of the material.[10]

An understanding of the foam-recovery or rebound-phenomenon properties of these materials has also led to recommendations in their use as shoe insoles. Both Pelite and Plastazote regain a percentage of their original thickness after removal of cyclic compressive loading.[2, 10] These findings have prompted the recommendations for an insole rotation procedure. This rotation procedure consists of issuing several pairs of insoles for daily changes to permit insoles compressed during a day's use sufficient time to recover in thickness during the interval of nonuse.[10]

Nonmoldable materials such as PPT (Langer Biomechanics Group, Inc., Deer Park, NY), Poron (ACOR Orthopaedic, Inc., Cleveland, OH), and the viscoelastic polymers Sorbothane (Sorbothane, Inc., Kent, OH) and Viscolas (Chattanooga Corp., Chattanooga, TN) are also widely used commercially available materials. Although there are distinct disadvantages to their lack of moldability, these materials resist shear-compression forces better than the polyethylene foams under controlled loading conditions.[2] Shock-absorbing and energy-return characteristics have been effectively demonstrated with PPT and Viscolas materials.[12, 17]

Leather and cork fall into the semirigid/semiflexible category of materials. Semirigid materials may be considered accommodative in their intended purpose, but they provide more functional support than soft materials and have longer life spans.[9] Many of the cork materials are now being combined with plastic compounds to make them moldable when heated. High-temperature thermoplastic polymers such as polypropylene and polyethylene, as well as the acrylic plastics and metals such as steel and aluminum alloys, are considered rigid materials. These materials offer the most support and durability. They are moldable at very high temperatures (300 to 400°F [149 to 204°C] or higher in some cases) and alter selected aspects of lower extremity kinematics. Polypropylene is one of the most widely adopted thermoplastic materials because its unique flexing properties enable it to withstand significant repetitive stress before showing signs of failure.[18] Polypropylene and polyethylene have been considered by some users to be semirigid when compared to their more rigid acrylic counterparts such as Rohadur (Glasflex, Stirling, NJ), or its replacements such as Flexidur (Active International, Hillside, NJ), and Polydor (Glasflex, Stirling, NJ).

Steel is also widely used in prefabricated joints, metal uprights, metal bands and cuffs, and springs and bearings of lower-limb orthoses. Steel is fatigue-resistant and combines high strength with high rigidity. The obvious disadvantage is its weight. The use of aluminum in orthoses is indicated when light weight is a major consideration. Although its static loading strength is good, aluminum has a lower endurance limit (or ability to withstand repetitive stress before failure) when compared to steel.[18] Therefore, if loading conditions are great and highly repetitive, as in the case of a large, active adult who ambulates with bilateral KAFOs, steel is preferred over aluminum.

As mentioned previously, the specific design and choice of materials vary according to the individual needs of the patient. Frequently, various materials are combined to achieve a desired outcome. Softer, accommodative materials may be selected for their shock absorption, total contact, and pressure distribution characteristics. They can be used in combination with semirigid or rigid materials for control, stabilization, and correction.[9] The need to develop thin, strong, and lightweight materials for orthotic construction has brought about the use of composite materials consisting of a combination of resin and graphite or fiberglass. The disadvantage of composites is that, once formed onto a positive cast, they are unable to be reshaped because of the nature of the thermosetting resin.[1] Should fitting problems arise, making adjustments is no longer possible.

For a complete list of suppliers of materials and equipment used in orthotics, the reader should consult the product index of the yearbook provided by the American Prosthetic and Orthotic Association available in medical libraries.

ADDITIONAL FACTORS IN THE CONSIDERATION OF ORTHOTIC APPLIANCES

In addition to the mechanical, prophylactic, and rehabilitative goals of orthotic intervention, other prescriptive considerations are equally important for achieving successful outcome. The sensitivity of the skin and underlying tissues must be known, for these factors may limit the magnitude and direction of forces that are applied to the skin. Orthotic prescription should take into account other biologic functions of the skin including skin integrity and cleanliness. Attention must be given to adequate ventilation and ease of cleaning the appliance, especially for the long-term user. Although orthotic use is not contraindicated in persons who have a loss of protective sensation or cognitive deficits, the selection of materials and their application over bony prominences warrant careful consideration.

There are other issues of concern in the prescription process. Increased physical demands and changes in energy expenditure need to be considered, particularly for the user with bilateral KAFOs.[26] Studies have shown that the rate of energy expenditure for individuals with paraplegia ambulating with bilateral KAFOs and using a swing-through gait pattern was 16.3 ml/kg/min.[25] In comparison, the rate was 6.3 ml/kg/min for able-bodied persons ambulating at the same speed. These findings represent an O_2 consumption rate 160% greater for those with paraplegia.

Orthoses should also be assessed for their effect on all levels of functional performance. This assessment should not be restricted to the impact of the orthosis on the performance of the athlete. The effect of the orthosis on transitional functional tasks such as sitting to standing, particularly for persons with neurologic or musculoskeletal deficits, is equally critical. Likewise, an awareness of the user's ability to put on or remove the appliance is essential, particularly if there is loss of upper extremity or trunk function.

Ideally, the orthotic prescription should incorporate a predictive component, or a "vision" for the future of the wearer. Changes in neurologic or musculoskeletal status need to be accompanied by a reassessment of the objectives and timely orthotic modifications. Given the unstable economic climate of health care reimbursement, cost undoubtedly will be a major concern that presents a challenge to providing effective orthotic management.

SUMMARY

Deciding which orthosis is best suited for a given individual is a complex process involving many different factors. The ability to successfully manage biomechanical abnormalities may be enhanced by an understanding of the properties of different orthotic materials, their effect on functional performance, and other associated patient factors. Health care providers are faced with the challenge of effectively addressing both the physiologic and the fiscal needs of the orthotic user in a rapidly changing health care environment.

REFERENCES

1. Berenter RW, Kosai DK: Various types of orthoses used in podiatry. Clin Podiatr Med Surg 11:219–229, 1994.
2. Brodsky JW, Kourosh S, Stills M, et al: Objective evaluation of insert material for diabetic and athletic footwear. Foot Ankle 9:111–116, 1988.
3. Burstein AH, Wright TM: Fundamentals of Orthopaedic Biomechanics, Baltimore, Williams & Wilkins, 1994, pp 137–140.
4. Byars EF, Snyder RD, Plants HL: Engineering Mechanics of Deformable Bodies, 4th ed, New York, Harper & Row Publishers, Inc., 1983, pp 224–237.
5. Eckhous D: Comparison of orthotic insert materials. Course manual, Prosthetics and Orthotics Course, Rancho Los Amigos Medical Center, 1985, pp 6–14.
6. Fuerbach JW, Grabiner MD, Koh TJ, et al: Effect of an ankle orthosis and ankle ligament anesthesia on ankle joint proprioception. Am J Sports Med 22:223–229, 1994.
7. Garcia AC, Dura JV, Ramiro J, et al: Dynamic study of insole materials simulating real loads. Foot Ankle Int 15:311–323, 1994.
8. Hewson GF, Mendini RA, Wang JB: Prophylactic knee bracing in college football. Am J Sports Med 14:262–266, 1986.

9. Janisse DJ: Indications and prescriptions for orthoses in sports. Orthop Clin North Am 25:95–107, 1994.
10. Kuncir EJ, Wirta RW, Golbranson FL: Load-bearing characteristics of polyethylene foam: An examination of structural and compression properties. J Rehabil Res Dev 27:229–238, 1990.
11. Leber C, Evanski PM: A comparison of shoe insole materials in plantar pressure relief. Prosthet Orthot Int 10:135–138, 1986.
12. Lewis G, Tan T, Shiue YS: Characterization of the performance of shoe insert materials. J Am Podiatr Med Assoc 81:418–424, 1991.
13. MacKean LC, Bell G, Burnham RS: Prophylactic ankle bracing versus taping: Effects on functional performance in female basketball players. J Orthop Sports Phys Ther 22:77–81, 1995.
14. Nawoczenski DA, Cook TM, Saltzman CL: The effect of foot orthotics on three-dimensional kinematics of the leg and rear foot during running. J Orthop Sports Phys Ther 21:317–327, 1995.
15. Nichols CE: Patellar tendon injuries. Clin Sports Med 11:807–812, 1992.
16. Palumbo PM: Dynamic patellar brace: A new orthosis in the management of patellofemoral disorders. Am J Sports Med 9:45–49, 1981.
17. Pratt DJ, Rees PH, Rodgers C: Assessment of some shock absorbing insoles. Prosthet Orthot Int 10:43–45, 1986.
18. Redford JB: Materials for orthotics. In Redford JB (ed): Orthotics Etcetera, 3rd ed, Baltimore, Williams & Wilkins, 1986, pp 58, 71.
19. Schultz AB, Hirsch C: Mechanical analysis techniques for improved correction of idiopathic scoliosis. Clin Orthop 100:66, 1974.
20. Sitler M, Ryan J, Wheeler B, et al: The efficacy of semi-rigid ankle stabilizer to reduce acute ankle injuries in basketball. Am J Sports Med 22:454–460, 1994.
21. Smith EM, Juvinall RC: Mechanics of orthotics. In Redford JB (ed): Orthotics Etcetera, 3rd ed, Baltimore, Williams & Wilkins, 1986, pp 26–32.
22. Surve I, Schwellness MD, Noakes T, et al: A five fold reduction in the incidence of recurrent ankle sprains on soccer players using the sport-stirrup orthoses. Am J Sports Med 22:601–605, 1994.
23. Thabit G, Micheli LJ: Patellofemoral pain in the pediatric patient. Orthop Clin North Am 23:567–585, 1992.
24. Tietz CC, Hermanson BK, Kronmal RA: Evaluation of the use of braces to prevent injury to the knee in college football players. J Bone Joint Surg 69A:2–9, 1987.
25. Waters RL, Lunsford BR: Energy cost of paraplegic ambulation. J Bone Joint Surg 67A, 1245, 1985.
26. Waters RL, Yakura JS: The energy expenditure of normal and pathological gait. Crit Rev Phys Med Rehabil 1:183–209, 1989.
27. White AA, Panjabi MM (eds): Clinical Biomechanics of the Spine, 2nd ed, Philadelphia, J.B. Lippincott Co., 1990, pp 348, 476, 505–506.

CHAPTER 2

Orthoses for the Pelvic and Hip Region

PETER J. MILLER

Orthotic intervention for the pelvic and hip regions does not span a wide range of physical dysfunctions, as it does in the remainder of the lower extremity. This chapter focuses on the use of orthotic systems for four different dysfunctions: low back pain of sacroiliac origin, total hip arthroplasty revisions, paraplegia, and functional hip orthoses. The mechanisms of action and effectiveness in clinical populations are also discussed.

SACROILIAC SUPPORT BELTS

Dysfunction of the sacroiliac joint has been implicated as a source of back pain by several authors.[1, 14, 18, 23, 26, 29] However, the prevalence of sacroiliac joint dysfunction has always been controversial. Some authors, such as Cyriax,[4] discount the possibility of sacroiliac joint subluxation causing pain, whereas others, such as Dontigny,[5] argue that sacroiliac joint dysfunction is a major cause of idiopathic low back pain. The lack of consensus regarding sacroiliac joint dysfunction may be due to two factors: the various descriptions of sacroiliac joint anatomy, biomechanics, and dysfunction,[1] and the difficulties associated with examining and diagnosing sacroiliac joint problems.

Vleeming et al[28] found that the sacroiliac joint surfaces can vary both in the coarseness of the articular cartilage and in the presence of ridges and depressions. These anatomic variations influence sacroiliac joint mobility.[29] Although it is now generally agreed that the sacroiliac joint does allow motion, Sturesson et al[26] found a mean of only 2.5 degrees of total rotation and 0.7 mm of total translation in a group of 25 patients with unilateral low back pain. They found no significant difference in the motion between symptomatic and asymptomatic sides.

Although a variety of nomenclature and descriptors exists, hypermobility and positional faults constitute the two general categories used to describe sacroiliac joint dysfunctions. Hypermobility of the sacroiliac joint is commonly associated with pregnancy[30] when the hormone relaxin increases the extensibility of the ligaments supporting the sacroiliac joint and the symphysis pubis. The stretched ligaments can become a source of pain as the superincumbent weight increases during the pregnancy. Hypermobility can also be caused by trauma.[30] Positional faults are characterized by sacroiliac joints that are "locked" in a position other than their normal resting position,[5] involving either anterior or posterior rotation of the ilium on the sacrum. Hypermobility and positional faults are not necessarily distinct entities; both Vleeming et al[29] and Edmond[6] describe how sacroiliac joint hypermobility can lead to a positional fault.

Understanding of sacroiliac joint dysfunction is further compromised by the inability of imaging technology (e.g., magnetic resonance imaging) to identify physical evidence that correlates with symptoms[23] and by the poor reliability of clinical tests of sacroiliac joint dysfunction.[21]

Rationale for Use and Mechanism of Action

Sacroiliac support belts have been recommended for use in the early stages of rehabilitation of lumbosacral spine dysfunctions[20] as a means to decrease pain and to provide mechanical support to the pelvis. Additionally, these belts have been recommended for use in soft tissue injuries of the pelvis and lumbosacral junction.[18]

Varying mechanisms of action have been proposed for sacroiliac support belts. The Lumbo-Pelvic Support (IEM Orthopaedic Systems, Inc., Ravenna, OH) consists of two straps joined posteriorly by a rigid trapezoid-shaped sacral pad that is thicker inferiorly than superiorly (Fig. 2–1). Porterfield and DeRosa[19] reported that this belt provides an anteroinferiorly directed force on the sacrum, facilitating sacral extension (counternutation), and a posterior rotation force of the ilia on the sacrum. The result is a posterior tilting force acting on the entire pelvis, which in turn decreases anterior shear forces created by superincumbent body weight at the lumbosacral junction. The authors also state that the support of the belt compresses the soft tissues surrounding the sacroiliac joints, thereby reducing the tensile stresses that are imposed on the tissues.

Porterfield and DeRosa[20] also offer a second mechanism of action for the sacroiliac support belt. Although the belt cannot completely immobilize the sacroiliac joints, the authors contend that it provides cutaneous input to the patient, which theoretically facilitates proprioceptive and kinesthetic awareness of spinal posture and movement. This awareness in turn would help the patient avoid positions and motions that could cause or aggravate sacroiliac joint symptoms.

A third proposed mechanism for sacroiliac support belt action is that it provides stability of the sacroiliac joints by reducing the amount of motion available.[33] The SI-LOC (OPTP, Minneapolis, MN) is a single fabric strap with anteriorly placed double Velcro closures (Fig. 2–2) that is purported by the manufacturer to approximate the two ilia closer together, thereby compressing the sacroiliac joints and the symphysis pubis. This mechanism

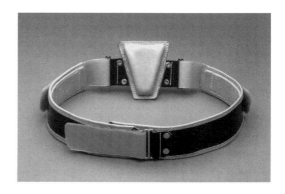

FIGURE 2–1. Lumbo-Pelvic Support with rigid sacral pad. (Courtesy of IEM Orthopaedic Systems, Inc., Ravenna, OH.)

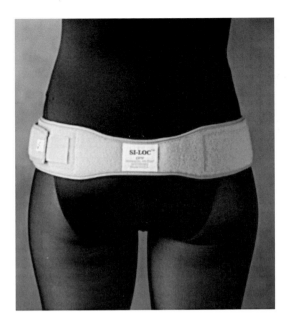

FIGURE 2-2. The SI-LOC (OPTP, Minneapolis, MN), a single fabric strap with double Velcro closures. (Courtesy of OPTP, Minneapolis, MN.)

of action would counteract the tendency of the superincumbent weight of the spinal column to separate the articular surfaces of the sacroiliac joint in that the wedge-shaped sacrum pushes the iliac bones apart. This type of belt may be indicated for patients who have sacroiliac joint symptoms secondary to hypermobility, but it may be inappropriate for patients who have positional faults of the sacroiliac joint, either anteriorly or posteriorly. For patients demonstrating positional faults of the sacroiliac joints, the increased compression provided by this belt would only make it more difficult to correct the positional fault and subsequently restore the normal joint position.

Another widely available sacroiliac support belt is the Sacroiliac Belt and Stabilization Pad (The Saunders Group, Chaska, MN). This support consists of a semirigid, elastic fabric belt that can be worn with or without a medium-density pad over the sacrum (Fig. 2–3). The manufacturer claims that the support offered by this belt works similarly to the mechanisms previously described that act to stabilize the sacrum and provide proprioceptive input to the patient. This support belt, as well as the aforementioned Lumbo-Pelvic Support, comes in a maternity version that features a wider, elastic anterior section of the belt (Fig. 2–4). These belts are designed to offer symptomatic relief to the expectant mother by stabilizing the sacroiliac joints against the hypermobility brought on by changes in hormonal activity and increased superincumbent weight.

To date, there is no scientific evidence to indicate that any sacroiliac support belt actually works by the mechanisms described. Alderink, in a

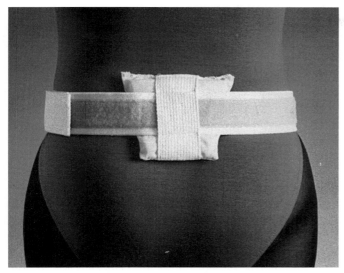

FIGURE 2–3. Sacroiliac Belt and Stabilization Pad (The Saunders Group, Chaska, MN) with removable medium-density sacral pad. (Courtesy of The Saunders Group, Chaska, MN.)

review of sacroiliac joint mechanics,[1] states that sacral movement is a product of superincumbent body weight and ground reaction forces. The question arises whether a support belt alone could produce opposing forces of sufficient magnitude to create sacral movement. Likewise, authors and manufacturers who report that the sacroiliac support belts cause compression and stabilization of the sacroiliac joints have offered no substantiating physical evidence for these claims. It is also possible that the compressive forces

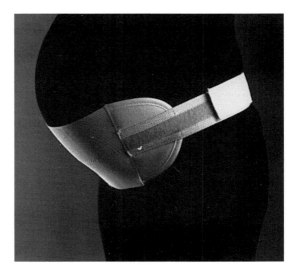

FIGURE 2–4. Maternity Sacroiliac Belt (The Saunders Group, Chaska, MN) features a wide anterior section. (Courtesy of The Saunders Group, Chaska, MN.)

caused by the tightness of the supports may be partly or totally absorbed by the soft tissues surrounding the pelvis, especially in obese or pregnant individuals, thereby limiting the action of the belts on the sacroiliac joint.

The mechanism of action that suggests the use of a support belt to provide proprioceptive/kinesthetic feedback may be valid. To date, however, there is no evidence to support that these belts alter either posture or movement in a patient population through this mechanism.

Effectiveness in Clinical Trials

The effectiveness of sacroiliac joint support belts in a patient population has not been well documented. Walheim[30] found that 11 out of 12 patients with clinical signs of pelvic instability experienced decreased pain when the joints were stabilized, but this stabilization was achieved with temporary external fixation devices. In a group of eight adult patients with unilateral sacroiliac joint dysfunction, as determined by clinical examination, Conway and Herzog[3] examined the changes in the magnitude of ground reaction forces when the patients were wearing a sacroiliac support belt. These investigators found no difference in the ground reaction forces when the patients walked with the support belt on compared to walking with the support belt off, or when walking with the support belt in a "placebo" position (that is, superior to the normal wearing position). The authors postulated that the support belt may have restricted sacroiliac movement, but they did not submit the data to statistical analysis.

Although evidence regarding the efficacy of sacroiliac support belts is lacking, many patients have experienced symptomatic relief and improved function when using the supports, and there have been no reports of negative effects. Subjective feedback appears to warrant their continued use, but a foundation of scientific knowledge about the biomechanical effects of sacroiliac support belts and the specific patient types that they would benefit is still needed.

TOTAL HIP REPLACEMENT ORTHOSES

More than 120,000 total hip replacements (THRs) are performed in the United States annually, and the National Institutes of Health Consensus Statement has concluded that THR is a successful treatment for hip dysfunction with an excellent prognosis for the patient.[27] The primary complication of a THR is loosening of the prosthetic components, which is believed to be caused by a massive osteolytic (bone resorption) reaction around the components.[27] Osteolysis can occur in both cemented and uncemented THRs and has been observed in up to 40% of THRs within 10 years of surgery.[27]

If loosening of the prosthetic components occurs, the patient may undergo total hip replacement revision surgery.[16, 27] The major complication of revision surgery is postoperative dislocation of the prosthetic hip joint. Dislocation, which has a reported incidence ranging from 0.5% to 5% in primary THR, ranges from 1% to 20% following revision surgery.[1, 14, 23, 26, 29] The most common direction of dislocation is posterior, which can be caused by excessive hip flexion, adduction, and internal rotation, and most dislocations occur within 6 weeks of the surgery.[17, 22] Prosthetic hip dislocations are associated with several factors, including surgical approach,[15, 22] component positioning,[22] improper patient positioning,[17] and patient noncompliance.[17, 22] The most startling statistic regarding prosthetic hip dislocation is presented by Blewitt and Mortimore,[2] who found that 65% of patients who suffered dislocations died within 6 months of the dislocation, presumably owing to the medical complications brought on by immobility.

Various treatment approaches have been used to decrease the incidence of dislocation, including the use of an anterior surgical approach, as opposed to the conventional posterior approach,[22] the use of a knee immobilizer to limit the patient's ability to flex or adduct the hip,[22] and the use of a modified hip spica cast.[17, 22] A postoperative hip orthosis has been used to decrease the incidence of dislocation.[16, 17, 25]

Rationale for Use and Mechanism of Action

The rationale for the use of a postoperative THR orthosis is to limit the hip motions (flexion, adduction, and internal rotation) that can cause dislocation. A commonly available version of the orthosis is the Newport Hip System (Orthomerica Products, Inc., Newport Beach, CA), which is a prefabricated, modular orthosis with an adjustable range-of-motion capability in two planes (Fig. 2–5). The orthosis can allow up to 70 degrees of hip flexion, with

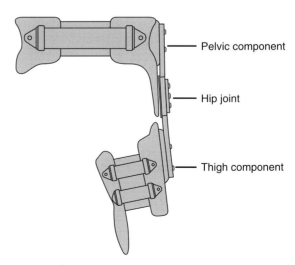

Pelvic component

Hip joint

Thigh component

FIGURE 2–5. Newport Hip System (Orthomerica Products, Inc., Newport Beach, CA) with a biaxial hip joint to allow 70 degrees of flexion, 0 degrees of extension, and 15 degrees of abduction, while preventing adduction beyond neutral. (Redrawn from Orthomerica Products, Inc., Newport Beach, CA.)

extension blocked at neutral. Frontal plane control is achieved by means of a joint that can be preset at 15 degrees of abduction or adjusted to other points in the abduction range. Adduction beyond neutral is not allowed in the orthosis. Rotational control of the lower extremity is maintained by the quality of the fit of the thigh component and can be enhanced by the addition of a lower leg component.

The orthosis is applied as early as the first or second postoperative day and is worn for 3 to 12 weeks following primary hip replacement or revision surgery.[13, 16]

Effectiveness in Clinical Trials

Stewart[25] examined the effect of a postoperative total hip orthosis in a group of 17 patients with THRs, four of whom had no history of dislocation and 13 of whom had at least one dislocation. Two patients (12%) experienced dislocation during the 3-month wearing period, and four more (24%) experienced dislocation after the wearing period ended. All the dislocations, except one, occurred in patients with a previous history of dislocation. Mallory et al[17] studied the effect of prophylactic use of a postoperative total hip orthosis in a group of 67 patients, of whom 30 underwent primary THR and 37 had revision surgery. Of the patients with revisions, three experienced dislocation within 6 months of the procedure. Each of these patients had undergone multiple revisions prior to the use of the orthosis. Of the primary THR patients, none suffered dislocation within 6 months of the surgery. The authors stated that the postrevision dislocation rate of 8% was an improvement over the previously reported incidence rate of 20%, but they did not use a control group in their research design to assess the significance of their findings. Lima et al[16] also studied the postrevision dislocation rate in a group of 80 patients who wore a postoperative hip orthosis for an average of 8 weeks. The investigators found that seven patients (8%) later experienced dislocation, although the follow-up period was not reported. Similar to the previous investigators, these authors did not compare their treatment group to a control group.

Although the use of a postoperative total hip orthosis may reduce the incidence of postrevision hip complications, dislocations can still occur. Lima et al[16] examined the characteristics of the seven subjects who experienced dislocation despite the use of the orthosis. The authors associated these dislocations with numerous factors, including a history of dislocations, poor hip abductor muscle strength, adductor spasticity, poor prosthetic positioning, and multiple prior operations.

The use of postoperative total hip orthoses appears to decrease the incidence of postrevision hip dislocation, but additional studies with a control group design are needed to verify the orthotic effectiveness for reducing the frequency of dislocation and to examine the influence on a patient's overall functional ability.

PARAPLEGIC ORTHOTIC WALKING SYSTEMS

Spinal cord injury or disease that causes paraplegia results not only in the loss of physical function, but also in the perceived loss of social and vocational abilities, especially in the early stages following the injury. Because most persons with paraplegia are young (mean age = 30 years), concerns arise regarding the likelihood of being able to stand and walk.[11] The ability to stand and walk is considered critical in the individual's potential to return to a normal lifestyle. Standing and walking offer many physiologic and psychological benefits to the person with paraplegia, and in the past 20 years there has been an increase in the research and development of rehabilitation technology, enabling more patients to stand and ambulate. It is now possible for persons with spinal cord lesions as high as T4 to ambulate.[24] Despite the improvements in orthotic intervention, however, standing and walking still present a major physical challenge for persons with paraplegia.

Rationale for Use

The ability of a person with paraplegia to stand upright imparts several positive physiologic effects, including improvement in circulation, reduction in spasticity, retardation of osteoporosis, prevention of joint contractures, and improvement in kidney function.[11] The achievement of successful paraplegic gait can also increase a person's functional ability in environments where wheelchair access is restricted or absent. In addition, the ability to stand and walk may confer psychological benefits to persons with paraplegia, as they may feel that this ability makes them more "abled" and part of the "normal" population.

Types of Devices

Although the most commonly used orthotic system for the paraplegic population is the bilateral knee-ankle-foot orthosis (KAFO), tremendous energy expenditure is required for the patient to walk.[24] The development of the hip-knee-ankle-foot orthosis (HKAFO) for paraplegic gait[11, 24] has allowed ambulation at a lower energy cost than that required with bilateral KAFOs.[9] This lower energy cost is permitted by the use of a reciprocal, step-through gait pattern, which most persons with paraplegia cannot attain with bilateral KAFOs because most of these orthoses require a nonreciprocal, swing-through pattern.

There are two major designs of HKAFOs. The Hip Guidance Orthosis (HGO), also known as the ORLAU ParaWalker, was developed in Oswestry, England, in 1979[8, 9, 12, 24, 31] (Fig. 2–6A). The Reciprocating Gait Orthosis (RGO), also known as the LSU Brace, was developed at Louisiana State

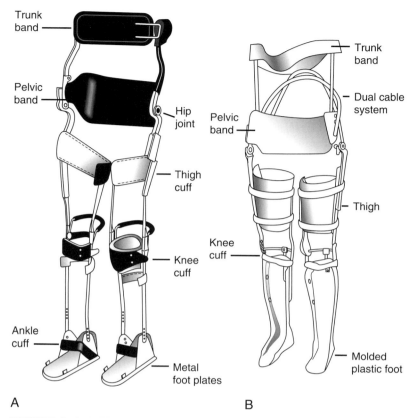

FIGURE 2-6. *A*, The Hip Guidance Orthosis (HGO). *B*, The Reciprocating Gait Orthosis (RGO).

University in 1983[9, 10, 12, 24, 31, 32] (Fig. 2–6*B*). These orthotic systems are similar in that the patient is braced from the mid-trunk level to the feet, with the knees and ankles immobilized in a neutral position. Both types of orthoses allow hip flexion and extension but prevent hip adduction.

The HGO and RGO also have several differences in design and function.[18] The HGO has a freely moving hip joint and metal foot plates that fit onto the outside soles of the patient's shoes. The HGO is worn outside the patient's clothes and can be used with axillary crutches. The RGO has a dual cable system that allows reciprocal hip flexion and extension between the contralateral orthotic hip joints, and it has a molded plastic foot section that fits inside the patient's shoes. The RGO is worn inside the patient's clothes and usually requires the use of a rolling or reciprocating walker. The HGO is heavier and less flexible, but easier to don than the RGO.

Two other HKAFOs derived from the RGO are available. The Steeper's Orthosis was developed in London, England in 1990[12] and is different from the RGO in that it uses a single cable system linking the two orthotic hip joints instead of a dual cable system. The Steeper's Orthosis also features spring mechanisms on the thigh components, which create a knee extension moment, allowing the patient to rise to standing from a sitting position in which the knees are flexed. Unlike the Steeper's Orthosis, the knee joints of the HGO and the RGO must be manually locked into extension prior to standing.

Another modification of the RGO is the Isocentric RGO, developed in Texas in 1992.[32] The Isocentric RGO replaces the cable system linking the orthotic hip joints with a centrally pivoting bar and tie rod arrangement, which is designed to be more energy-efficient than the cable system.

Mechanisms of Action

Regardless of the type of design, the HKAFOs used for paraplegic gait have a similar mechanism of action.[12] The patient stands with the ankles locked in neutral position and the knees locked in full extension. Hip control is managed by trunk and arm stabilization, along with upper-extremity weight bearing on an assistive device. Some patients can stand successfully without an assistive device.[32] Ambulation is achieved by advancing the assistive device, which results in flexion of the trunk. The patient then hikes the pelvis on the side of the trailing leg, which allows the trailing leg to swing forward. This pattern is then repeated to advance the opposite lower extremity. In the HGO design, the hips are freely moving in the plane of flexion and extension (although there are built-in motion stops). The RGO (as well as its modifications) is designed so that the two linked hips cause reciprocal motion, in that extension on one side causes flexion on the other. Ferrarin et al[8] studied the kinematic and kinetic parameters of gait in patients with paraplegia who used an HGO. They found that the more experienced the patient was with the HGO, the more the gait pattern progressed from being a series of interrupted steps to a more fluid, continuous pattern.

Effectiveness in Clinical Trials

Whittle et al[31] compared the effectiveness and use of the HGO and RGO in a population of 22 patients with complete paraplegia. Each patient was given the option to use either orthosis for 4 months. Of the 22 patients, 15 used both orthoses, two preferred the HGO over the RGO, and five did not use either orthosis for any extensive period. The patients reported that both systems needed frequent adjustments and that the skin had to be monitored closely, especially with the RGO, which is worn against the skin. The subjects found that rising from sitting to standing was easier with the RGO, and that walking over functional distances was easier with the RGO and a rolling walker than with the HGO and axillary crutches.

Jefferson and Whittle[12] compared the kinematics of gait in a single paraplegic subject with a complete T6 lesion who wore the HGO, the RGO, and the Steeper's Orthosis in a laboratory setting. The subject used crutches when ambulating with the HGO and a rolling walker when ambulating with the RGO and the Steeper's Orthosis. Although the stride length was the same for all three orthoses, findings indicated that different amounts of range of motion occurred in the hips. The authors were unable to differentiate whether these range-of-motion differences were due to the orthoses or due to the combined effect of the orthoses and type of assistive device used.

Winchester et al[32] compared the energy cost of ambulating with the RGO to the energy cost with the Isocentric RGO in four patients with complete paraplegia (level not reported). The results indicated a lower energy cost with the Isocentric RGO as compared to the standard RGO, but the sample size was too small to make any definitive conclusions.

Despite advances in rehabilitation engineering, achieving a practical, efficient form of standing and walking has proven to be an elusive goal for most persons with paraplegia. The other major development in paraplegic gait has been the use of functional electrical stimulation (FES) to recruit the proper lower-extremity muscles in a gait-appropriate sequence and magnitude. However, FES used alone has so far been of marginal benefit.[7, 10, 12] This finding results from the difficulty of achieving the proper stimulation parameters and programming, the difficulty of use, and system reliability. However, some research has indicated that a hybrid FES-orthosis system may be of some benefit. Hirokawa et al[9] found that ambulating with a system combining FES with an RGO required less energy expenditure than use of the RGO alone, in a sample of six individuals with paraplegic lesions from T1 to T10. Isakov et al[10] found that an FES-RGO system lowered the energy cost for rising to standing and for walking, compared to the RGO alone, for a patient with a complete T4 lesion.

Several factors determine the ultimate success of paraplegic gait with the orthotic systems described previously. These factors include the energy cost; the reliability of the device; cosmesis; safety; ease of donning and doffing; the cost of fabrication, training, service; and, of course, the level of independence afforded.[9, 24] The major drawback to the use of mechanical orthotic systems for paraplegic gait continues to be the tremendous energy expenditure for ambulation, which has been measured to be 5 to 12 times greater than that required for normal gait.[11]

Although it is understandable that many persons with paraplegia would prefer to walk during everyday activities, the use of a wheelchair is frequently the most practical, functional mode of locomotion. Wheelchairs are more energy-efficient and allow persons with paraplegia to travel faster. Although continued research and development of orthotic walking systems are necessary for persons with paraplegia, wheelchair accessibility in work and social environments must keep pace with this development.

FUNCTIONAL HIP ORTHOSES

Hip pointers, as well as muscular strains and contusions about the hip region, have traditionally been managed using various wraps and fabricated padding (see Chap. 7). Recent advances in the area of functional hip orthoses have provided a means to more easily and cost-effectively protect the hip region from reinjury or exacerbation of an already existing injury.

Rationale for Use and Mechanism of Action

Because the rationale for use and the mechanism of action are similar to those described in the use of wraps and fabricated protective padding, the reader is referred to the descriptions found in Chapter 7.

Sully Hip S'port

The Sully Hip S'port (The Saunders Group, Chaska, MN) is a functional hip orthosis comprised of Velcro-sensitive shorts that allow for attachment of neoprene support straps or a closed-cell foam pad at various locations on the shorts (Fig. 2–7). These neoprene straps can be positioned to effectively limit the excursion of hip movement in cases of muscular strains. Additionally, the foam pad can be applied for protection over areas of bruises and hip pointers.

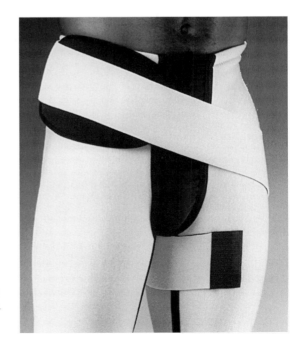

FIGURE 2–7. Sully Hip S'port (The Saunders Group, Chaska, MN) features Velcro-sensitive shorts for selective attachment of support straps and/or foam pads. (Courtesy of The Saunders Group, Chaska, MN.)

SUMMARY

This chapter described the rationale, mechanisms, and clinical effectiveness of four currently used orthotic devices for the pelvis and hip. Although the theoretical benefits of these devices are apparent, any real effectiveness can be supported only by scientific evidence. A comparison of the research testing for sacroiliac support belts, total hip replacement orthoses, and paraplegic orthotic walking systems shows an ascending level of research sophistication for the three devices. This finding may be due in part to the different levels of technical complexity of the devices, but even a very simple orthosis, such as the sacroiliac support belt, requires careful scientific inquiry to support its use as a clinical tool.

REFERENCES

1. Alderink GJ: The sacroiliac joint: Review of anatomy, mechanics, and function. J Orthop Sports Phys Ther 13:71–84, 1991.
2. Blewitt N, Mortimore S: Outcome of dislocation after hemiarthroplasty for fractured neck of the femur. Injury 23:320–322, 1992.
3. Conway PJ, Herzog W: Changes in walking mechanics associated with wearing an intertrochanteric support belt. J Manip Physiol Ther 14:185–188, 1991.
4. Cyriax J: Textbook of Orthopaedic Medicine. Vol 1, Diagnosis of Soft Tissue Lesions, 8th ed, London, Bailliere Tindall, 1978.
5. Dontigny RL: Anterior dysfunction of the sacroiliac joint as a major factor in the etiology of idiopathic low back pain syndrome. Phys Ther 70:250–262, 1990.
6. Edmond SL: Manipulation and Mobilization. Extremity and Spinal Techniques, St. Louis, Mosby-Year Book, 1993, pp 269–270.
7. Ewins DJ, Taylor PN, Lipczynski RT, et al: Practical low cost stand/sit system for mid-thoracic paraplegics. J Biomed Eng 10:184–188, 1988.
8. Ferrarin M, Pedotti A, Boccardi S, et al: Biomechanical assessment of paraplegic locomotion with hip guidance orthosis (HGO). Clin Rehabil 7:303–308, 1993.
9. Hirokawa S, Grimm M, Le T, et al: Energy consumption in paraplegic ambulation using the reciprocating gait orthosis and electric stimulation of the thigh muscles. Arch Phys Med Rehabil 71:687–694, 1990.
10. Isakov E, Douglas R, Berns P: Ambulation using the reciprocating gait orthosis and functional electrical stimulation. Paraplegia 30:239–245, 1992.
11. Jaeger RJ, Yarkony GM, Roth EJ: Rehabilitation technology for standing and walking after spinal cord injury. Am J Phys Med Rehabil 68:128–133, 1989.
12. Jefferson RJ, Whittle MW: Performance of three walking orthoses for the paralysed: a case study using gait analysis. Prosthet Orthot Int 14:103–110, 1990.
13. Kisner C, Colby LA: Therapeutic Exercise. Foundations and Techniques, 2nd ed, Philadelphia, F.A. Davis Co., 1990, pp 336–342.
14. LeBlanc KE: Sacroiliac sprain: An overlooked cause of back pain. Am Fam Physician 46:1459–1463, 1992.
15. Lewis CB, Knortz KA: Orthopedic Assessment and Treatment of the Geriatric Patient. St. Louis, Mosby-Year Book, 1993, pp 217–262.
16. Lima D, Magnus R, Paprosky WG: Team management of hip revision patients using a post-op hip orthosis. J Prosthet Orthot 6:20–24, 1994.
17. Mallory TH, Vaughn BK, Lombardi AV, et al: Prophylactic use of a hip cast-brace following primary and revision total hip arthroplasty. Orthop Rev 17:178–183, 1988.
18. Porterfield JA: Dynamic stabilization of the trunk. J Orthop Sports Phys Ther 6:271–277, 1985.

19. Porterfield JA, DeRosa C: Lumbar spine and pelvis. In Richardson JK, Iglarsh ZA (ed): Clinical Orthopaedic Physical Therapy, Philadelphia, W.B. Saunders Co., 1994, pp 119–158.
20. Porterfield JA, DeRosa C: Mechanical Low Back Pain. Perspectives in Functional Anatomy, Philadelphia, W.B. Saunders Co., 1991, pp 177–180.
21. Potter NA, Rothstein JM: Intertester reliability for selected clinical tests of the sacroiliac joint. Phys Ther 65:1671–1675, 1985.
22. Rao JP, Bronstein R: Dislocations following arthroplasties of the hip. Incidence, prevention, and treatment. Orthop Rev 20:261–264, 1991.
23. Schwarzer AC, Aprill CN, Bogduk N: The sacroiliac joint in chronic low back pain. Spine 20:31–37, 1995.
24. Stallard J, Major RE, Patrick JH: A review of the fundamental design problems of providing ambulation for paraplegic patients. Paraplegia 27:70–75, 1989.
25. Stewart HD: The hip cast-brace for hip prosthesis instability. Ann R Coll Surg Engl 65:404–406, 1983.
26. Sturesson B, Selvik G, Uden A: Movements of the sacroiliac joints. A roentgen stereophotogrammetric analysis. Spine 14:162–165, 1989.
27. Total Hip Replacement. NIH Consensus Statement, 12(5):1–31, Sep 12–14, 1994.
28. Vleeming A, Stoeckart R, Volkers AC, et al: Relation between form and function in the sacroiliac joint. Part I: Clinical anatomical aspects. Spine 15:130–132, 1990.
29. Vleeming A, Volkers AC, Snijders CJ, et al: Relation between form and function in the sacroiliac joint. Part II: Biomechanical aspects. Spine 15:133–135, 1990.
30. Walheim GG: Stabilization of the pelvis with the Hoffman frame. Acta Orthop Scand 55:319–324, 1984.
31. Whittle MW, Cochrane GM, Chase AP, et al: A comparative trial of two walking systems for paralysed people. Paraplegia 29:97–102, 1991.
32. Winchester PK, Carollo JJ, Parekh RN, et al: A comparison of paraplegic gait performance using two types of reciprocating gait orthoses. Prosthet Orthot Int 17:101–106, 1993.
33. Zohn DA: Musculoskeletal Pain, Diagnosis and Physical Treatment, 2nd ed, Boston, Little, Brown and Co, 1988, pp 158–159.

CHAPTER 3

Orthoses for the Knee: The Patellofemoral Joint

BARBARA C. BELYEA

"It seems likely that more has been written about the patella, relative to its size, than about any other bone in the human body."[11] This quotation by Haxton in 1945 still holds true in today's medical literature, as a plethora of research describes the clinical presentation and etiologic factors related to patellofemoral dysfunction. Although the symptoms and physical findings may be well documented, treatment approaches are still a source of controversy for health care providers. Diagnoses of these dysfunctions include patellofemoral pain syndrome, patellar subluxation and dislocation, patellar tendinitis, chondromalacia patellae, and arthritis due to degenerative changes occurring at the joint. The purposes of this chapter are to review the anatomy and biomechanical factors related to patellofemoral dysfunction to present the common clinical profiles associated with each of the pathologic conditions, and to discuss the various orthotic interventions and their clinical effectiveness in the treatment of these dysfunctions.

ANATOMY AND BIOMECHANICS OF THE PATELLOFEMORAL JOINT

Judged to be the least congruent joint in the body,[45] the patellofemoral joint consists of the articulation between the patella and the intercondylar groove on the anterior surface of the distal femur (Fig. 3–1). The patella, a triangularly shaped sesamoid bone with a proximal base and distal apex,[21] communicates with the common tendon of the quadriceps muscle.[31] Little variation has been found in the width and length of patellae, which range from 51 to 57 mm and 47 to 58 mm, respectively.[17] The posterior surface of the patella is covered with a thick layer of hyaline cartilage. The superior portion of this surface has a vertical ridge that divides the patella into medial and lateral facets that articulate with the femur (Fig. 3–2).[45] A second vertical ridge separates the medial facet from the odd facet, which articulates with the medial femoral condyle at full knee flexion.

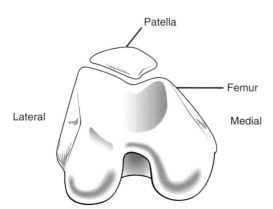

FIGURE 3–1. Articulating surfaces of the posterior patella and anterior femur.

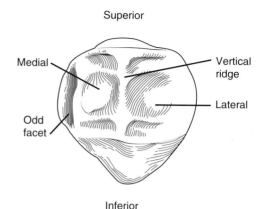

FIGURE 3–2. Articulating surface of the patella, divided into medial and lateral facets by a vertical ridge. Note the odd facet on the medial aspect of the patella.

The articulating surface of the distal femur consists of a groove that separates the medial and lateral femoral condyles (Fig. 3–3).[45] The vertical ridge of the patella communicates with the intercondylar groove of the femur. The anterior orientation of the lateral femoral condyle provides stability against lateral patellar displacement, which will be discussed later in this chapter.

The muscular component at the knee, referred to as the extensor mechanism, is composed of the four muscles of the quadriceps femoris: the rectus femoris, the vastus intermedius, the vastus lateralis, and the vastus medialis (Fig. 3–4). The extensor mechanism functions to extend the knee and contracts eccentrically to decelerate the knee during gait.[21] The four portions of the quadriceps muscle converge proximally to the patella to form the quadriceps tendon, which continues distally as the patellar tendon, and insert on the tibial tubercle.[45] Fibers from the vastus medialis and lateralis insert at various angles onto the medial and lateral aspects of the patella, respectively (Fig. 3–5). The vastus medialis oblique has a more sharply angled insertion of approximately 65 degrees.[21] These muscles play an im-

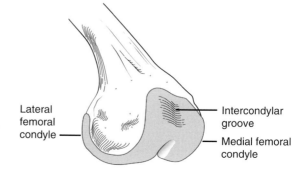

FIGURE 3–3. The intercondylar groove of the femur separates the medial and lateral femoral condyles and articulates with the vertical ridge of the patella.

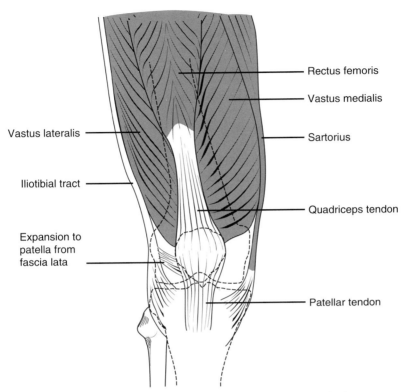

FIGURE 3-4. Structures comprising the extensor mechanism of the knee.

portant role in the static and dynamic positions and mediolateral stability of the patella.

The patella functions as an anatomic pulley to increase the lever arm of the quadriceps, thereby increasing its line of pull and improving the mechanical advantage of this primary knee extensor muscle group.[31, 45] The significance of this increase in muscle force is evidenced by the loss of up to 30% of torque output in the quadriceps following patellectomy.[45] The patella also absorbs the compressive forces imparted on the femur and prevents excessive friction on the quadriceps tendon.[17, 21] In order to perform its role properly, the patella must be able to slide or "track" appropriately in the intercondylar groove. The position of the patella and its ability to correctly track are controlled by both static and dynamic factors.

Variations in the shape and size of the facets (Fig. 3–6A) and depth of the intercondylar groove (referred to as the sulcus angle in Fig. 3–6B) can affect the stability and tracking of the patella.[21] As indicated in Figure 3–6A, six types of patellar configurations have been described.[61] Type I has relatively equal concave facets, whereas type II demonstrates a slightly smaller medial facet. The remaining classifications of patellae present with variations in the

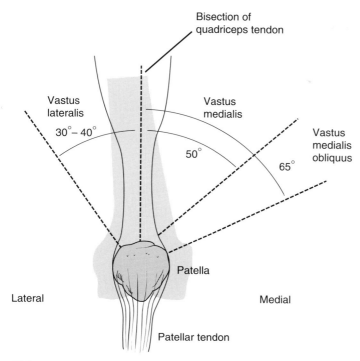

FIGURE 3–5. Schematic representation of the angles of insertion of the muscles of the extensor mechanism on the patella.

slope of the facets and depth of the central ridge. These variations can result in an uneven distribution of forces and unequal stresses on the articular surfaces. Therefore, patellae with relatively symmetric facets and articulating with deeper intercondylar grooves are the most stable. Conversely, asymmetric patellar facets articulating with shallower intercondylar grooves result in uneven distribution of compression forces and subsequent joint instability.

Other static structures providing stability to the patella include the medial and lateral retinacula and the joint capsule (Fig. 3–7). The lateral retinaculum consists of fibers that run from the iliotibial band to the patella. These bands become taut with knee flexion and tilt the patella laterally. This force is countered by the pull from the medial retinaculum bands.[17] Imbalances in the integrity of these structures can affect the position and kinematics of the patellofemoral joint.

Dynamic control of patellar tracking is achieved primarily by the quadriceps femoris muscle. Contraction of the quadriceps femoris causes knee extension, during which the patella glides superiorly in the intercondylar groove. With knee flexion, the patella glides inferiorly. For appropriate patellar tracking to occur, there must be a "balance" in the activity between the vastus medialis oblique and vastus lateralis. Purported imbalances be-

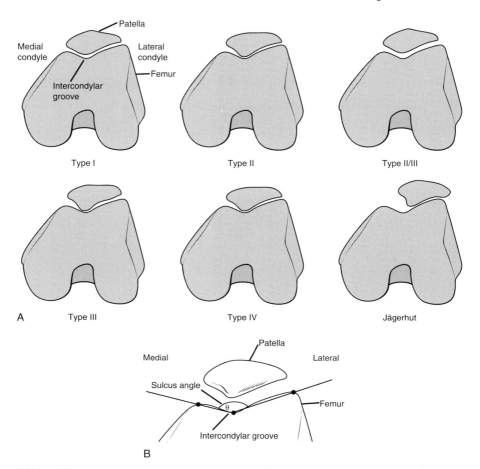

FIGURE 3–6. Variations in articular surfaces can affect the distribution of forces at the patellofemoral joint. *A*, Six classifications of patellar configurations, with varying degrees of depth and slopes of facets. *B*, Depth of the intercondylar groove influences the contact between the femur and the patella.

tween these two muscle groups may result in abnormal patellar alignment and maltracking, which may result in pain and degenerative changes in the articular cartilage.[39] Additional muscles that play a role in patellar stability through their attachments to the joint capsule include the gastrocnemius, semimembranosus, semitendinosus, iliotibial tract, and sartorius.[21]

Another factor contributing to patellar tracking is the Q angle. Formed by the line of pull of the quadriceps and the patellar tendon (Fig. 3–8), the Q angle normally ranges from 10 to 15 degrees.[45] Gender differences have been found in Q angle measurements, with the angle in males ranging from 10 to 12 degrees and in females ranging from 15 to 18 degrees.[20] Larger Q angles may be associated with increased femoral anteversion, excessive exter-

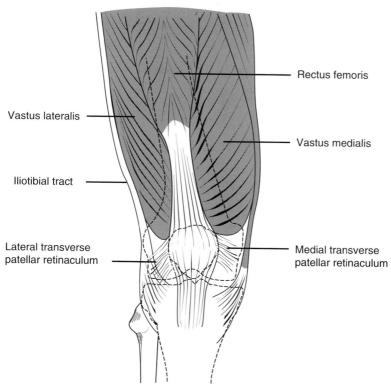

FIGURE 3-7. The medial and lateral retinacula and the joint capsule provide stability to the patella.

nal tibial torsion, or relative genu valgum, and they result in excessive lateral forces on the patella.[20, 45] Larger- or smaller-than-normal Q angles can create unpredictable patterns of cartilage loading and can present the potential for development of patellofemoral abnormalities.[26] Some authors, however, have cautioned against placing too much emphasis on the Q angle measurement. The static Q angle measurement that is assessed at full knee extension can change dramatically throughout the range of motion and during functional activity,[63] thereby limiting its full diagnostic significance.

The position of the patella in the femoral groove and the forces imparted on the joint, referred to as patellofemoral joint reaction (PFJR) forces, vary throughout knee range of motion (Table 3–1). At full knee extension, the patella "sits" in the intercondylar groove, making very little contact with the femur, and therefore exerts little to no compressive force.[45] As the knee flexes to about 10 to 20 degrees, the medial and lateral facets of the patella come into contact with the femur. The pull from the quadriceps tendon and from the patellar tendon compresses the patella into the femur, thereby increasing the joint reaction force. With increasing flexion up to 90 degrees,

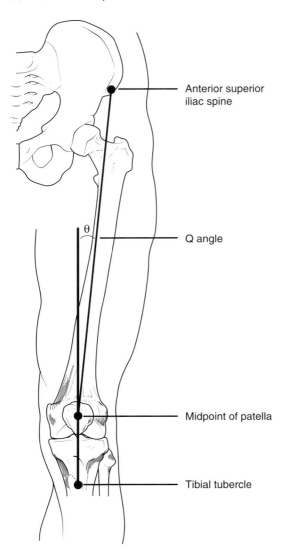

Anterior superior
iliac spine

Q angle

Midpoint of patella

Tibial tubercle

FIGURE 3–8. The Q angle,
formed by a line connecting the
anterior superior iliac spine to the
midpoint of the patella and a line
connecting the tibial tubercle and
the midpoint of the patella, influences patellar alignment and
tracking.

the PFJR force increases along with an increase in the articular surface area
of contact between the patella and femur. Greater contact area disperses the
increased force and maintains a relatively constant load on the joint structures.[17] Maximum contact force occurs at 90 degrees of flexion and approxi-
mates up to 6.5 times body weight.[26] As flexion continues past 90 degrees,
the patella rotates medially so that the ridge between the medial facet and
odd facet comes in contact with the medial femoral condyle. At 135 degrees
of knee flexion, the contact pressure is primarily located on the odd facet
and the lateral facet.[19, 21, 45] Throughout knee motion, the medial aspect of

TABLE 3–1

Comparison of the Patellar Position and Posterior Patellar Surface Area

Knee Joint Angle	Patellar Position	Patellofemoral Joint Reaction Forces	Patellar Surface Contact	
0°		—		Little to no contact
10–20°		↑		Medial and lateral facets with femoral groove
90°		↑		Medial and lateral facets, proximal patella, and odd facet
>90°		↓		Odd facet along medial femoral condyle

the patella receives the most contact, accounting for the increased frequency of degenerative changes in the cartilage at the medial and odd facets.[45]

In addition to joint position, the PFJR forces can be affected by the amount of active and passive pull of the quadriceps.[45] Between initial contact and loading response during gait, the PFJR force is approximately half of body weight, and it may increase to as much as 3.3 times body weight with stair climbing or running.[28] Compressive forces during cycling are approximately 1.5 times body weight.[15] Activities in extremes of knee flexion, which require strong quadriceps contraction (i.e., deep knee bends), may produce PFJR forces as high as 7.8 times body weight.[45] An understanding of these forces is essential when developing rehabilitation programs for people with patellofemoral joint dysfunctions.

MOVEMENT DYSFUNCTIONS AT THE PATELLOFEMORAL JOINT

The following section discusses the movement dysfunctions and clinical presentations associated with the most common patellofemoral dysfunctions. These pathologic conditions include patellofemoral pain syndrome (PFPS) (also referred to as anterior knee pain or patellar malalignment syndrome), patellar subluxation and dislocation, patellar tendinitis, and arthritic changes resulting in chondromalacia patellae.

Patellofemoral Pain Syndrome

One of the most common pathologic conditions involving the patellofemoral joint is PFPS.[21] The prevalence of PFPS has been shown to be as high as one in four in the athletic population,[33] and is reported to affect over 25% of recruits in military service.[60] In one study of 83 runners treated for knee complaints, 57.5% were diagnosed with PFPS.[56] The female-to-male ratio was found to be 3:2 by Goodfellow et al,[19] 2:1 by Gerrard,[18] and 2:3 by DeHaven et al.[10] Symptoms are common in early adolescence during growth spurts and may be related to imbalances in the muscles that provide medial and lateral stability at the patella.[22] The most common complaint associated with PFPS is anterior knee pain,[10] which is aggravated by stair climbing, prolonged sitting, and strenuous activity. Other symptoms include swelling, joint clicking, and a sensation of "giving way."[6, 10, 22] Clinical findings include painful patellar facets, excessive subtalar joint pronation, tight iliotibial bands, decreased eccentric torque production,[2] and reproduction of symptoms while performing the patellofemoral grinding test (Clarke's test) (Fig. 3–9).[10, 39]

The primary etiologic factor causing patellofemoral pain is abnormal stress imposed on the articular surface of the patella as a result of malalignment and maltracking.[29, 53] Malalignment may be the result of one or more

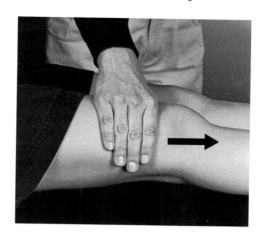

FIGURE 3–9. Clarke's test: Pain and crepitus are reproduced when a distal force is applied by the examiner to the superior patella during an isometric contraction of the quadriceps.

of the following factors: abnormal patellofemoral articulation, soft tissue deficiencies, and malalignment of the lower extremity.[31] Abnormalities between the patella and the femoral articular surfaces may also result from various anomalies, one of which is an increased sulcus angle. As previously discussed, the sulcus angle is the angle formed by the lateral and medial facets on the femur (see Fig. 3–6*B*). A greater angle results in a shallower intercondylar groove, creating patellar instability and potential maltracking. Another articular condition that may predispose an individual to maltracking is the vertical location of the patella relative to the femoral sulcus.[45] Normal positioning between the patella and femoral sulcus yields a 1:1 ratio of the length of the patellar tendon to the length of the patella. An excessively long tendon relative to patellar length results in a high-riding patella, known as patella alta (Fig. 3–10). A shortened patella tendon relative to patella length is referred to as patella baja, which may result in anterior knee pain due to increased patellofemoral contact forces.[21]

Soft tissue dysplasia is another major factor in PFPS. As previously discussed, the medial and lateral fibers of the quadriceps muscle, along with fibers from the iliotibial band, provide dynamic stability at the patella (Fig. 3–11). Imbalances in these soft tissue structures may result in patellar malalignment. One of the most commonly proposed theories of muscle imbalance is associated with poor control of the vastus medialis oblique (VMO). This condition results from muscle atrophy or slow recruitment of muscle fibers. Insufficiency of the VMO limits the potential of the muscle to equally oppose the pull of the vastus lateralis and lateral retinaculum, resulting in a laterally oriented patella.[3, 31, 39, 59] The consequences of this lateral orientation include abnormal patellar tracking in the intercondylar groove with increased compression on the lateral articular surfaces, leading to degenerative changes in the articular cartilage and pain.[58] In addition to VMO insufficiency, lateral patellar orientation may be related to an abnormally tight lateral retinacu-

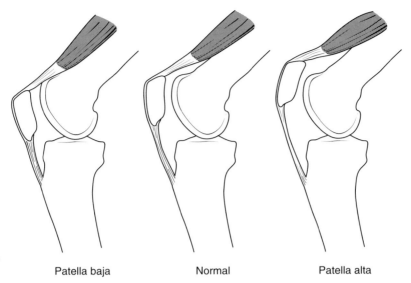

| Patella baja | Normal | Patella alta |

FIGURE 3–10. Patella baja and patella alta are examples of positional faults of the patella relative to the femoral sulcus. Normal positioning of the patella yields a 1:1 ratio of the length of the patellar tendon to the length of the patella.

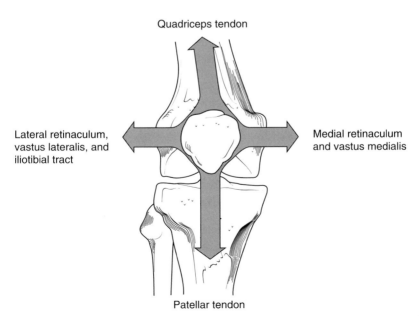

Quadriceps tendon

Lateral retinaculum, vastus lateralis, and iliotibial tract

Medial retinaculum and vastus medialis

Patellar tendon

FIGURE 3–11. Dynamic stability of the patella is affected by the length and strength contributions of the vastus medialis, vastus lateralis, and iliotibial band.

lum or iliotibial band, which places tension on the lateral border of the patella thereby causing it to tilt laterally.[31, 39]

Structural alignments of the lower extremity can also affect the orientation and tracking of the patella. As discussed previously, PFPS has been associated with an increased Q angle (see Fig. 3–8).[42] James et al[30] documented that 42% of patients with PFPS had Q angles greater than 20 degrees. Increased angles may be related to a wider pelvis, increased femoral anteversion, and excessive external tibial torsion.[45] The result is a relative shortening of the fibers of the vastus lateralis and a lengthening of the VMO fibers, rendering them inherently weaker and increasing the pressure on the lateral patellofemoral articular surfaces.[31]

Correlation has also been shown between PFPS and foot alignment.[1, 4, 6, 30, 42, 51, 58] Of particular concern are the amount and timing of subtalar joint pronation during the stance phase of gait (Fig. 3–12). Excessive subtalar joint pronation may cause excessive tibial internal rotation as well as delay the normal external rotation of the tibia. The changes in rotation may cause increased contact pressures between the lateral articular surfaces at the patellofemoral joint.[4, 6, 51, 58] In addition, if pronation occurs too soon in the gait cycle, the rearfoot is unable to dissipate the ground reaction forces. The patellofemoral joint then absorbs more force than usual, causing abnormal cartilage irritation and degeneration.[42]

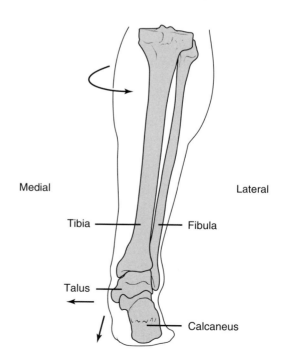

Medial

Lateral

Tibia

Fibula

Talus

Calcaneus

FIGURE 3–12. Alterations in the magnitude and timing of subtalar joint pronation may adversely impact the patellofemoral joint through the kinematic coupling between the foot and the leg.

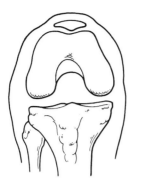 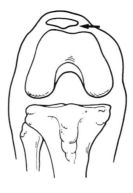

FIGURE 3–13. Patellar subluxation or dislocation usually occurs in a lateral direction. The patella may be pulled laterally out of the intercondylar groove as a result of structural instability or excessive pull generated by the lateral structures. (From Richardson JK, Iglarsh ZA: Clinical Orthopaedic Physical Therapy, Philadelphia, W.B. Saunders Co., 1994.)

Subluxation/Dislocation

Patellofemoral instability and excessive lateral pull on the patella can result in subluxation or dislocation of the patella from the intercondylar groove (Fig. 3–13). Subluxation and dislocations may result from progressive abnormal tracking due to lack of dynamic stability, or acute trauma in which a sudden change of direction is associated with a strong, decelerating contraction of the quadriceps.[6, 27] The surrounding structures frequently heal with less tensile strength, predisposing the patella to recurrent episodes of subluxation and dislocation.[27] Symptoms are similar to those of PFPS, including complaints of "giving way" at the knee, a feeling of the patella's slipping, and joint effusion.[24] Clinical evaluation typically reveals patella alta, lateral patellar tilt, VMO atrophy, lateral patellar hypermobility at 45 degrees of knee flexion, and apprehension with lateral patellar displacement (Fig. 3–14).[24, 27] Other physical findings may include genu valgum, genu recurvatum, forefoot pronation, and excessive femoral neck anteversion.[50]

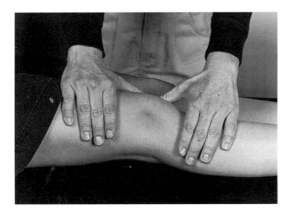

FIGURE 3–14. Lateral apprehension test: The patient exhibits signs of apprehension when a lateral glide of the patella is applied by the examiner. The test is indicative of lateral patellar subluxation or dislocation.

Patellar Tendinitis

Tendinitis is defined as the inflammation of a tendon in response to injury. The source of injury in most cases of tendinitis is a chronic overuse that places repeated stress on the tendon, causing microtearing of the collagen fibers.[8, 38, 52] Patellar tendinitis, also referred to as "jumper's knee," is an inflammation of the patellar tendon and is commonly seen in athletes who perform forceful jumping or kicking movements such as those used in basketball, volleyball, and soccer.[52] Although inflammation may occur anywhere along the patellar tendon, the most common site is at the attachment to the inferior patellar pole (Fig. 3–15).[8] At this location, the tendon narrows and assumes a large concentration of stress during explosive knee extension. The site of irritation along the tendon may also vary with age. Inflammation at the insertion of the tibial tubercle is most common in growing children, whereas involvement at the apex of the patella is more common in people over 40 years of age.[8]

The most common complaint in cases of patellar tendinitis is infrapatellar pain and point tenderness, aggravated during eccentric quadriceps contraction.[8] Patients may also report stiffness with prolonged knee flexion. Clinical findings may include patellar hypermobility, quadriceps atrophy, patellar malalignment, and hamstring tightness.[44] Radiography is usually inconclusive, except in the case of Osgood-Schlatter disease, which is a traction apophysitis of the tibial tubercle resulting from continued stress on a weakened patellar tendon (see Fig. 3–15).[5]

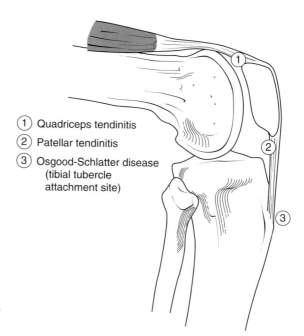

① Quadriceps tendinitis
② Patellar tendinitis
③ Osgood-Schlatter disease
  (tibial tubercle
  attachment site)

FIGURE 3–15. Common sites of inflammation and irritation of the tendinous structures.

Articular Cartilage Lesions/Patellar Arthrosis

Several medical authors have debated the relationship between degenerative changes in the articular cartilage at the patellofemoral joint and patellar pain.[17, 20, 22, 29] The link between patellar arthrosis and symptomatic knees is questionable. Many patients with asymptomatic knees have extensive degenerative changes; conversely, symptomatic knees often do not reveal true morphologic changes.

Chondromalacia patellae, or softening of the cartilage, has been a widely used diagnosis referring to any case of anterior knee pain regardless of the presence of actual articular changes. In accordance with recent literature, the term chondromalacia patellae is used in this text to refer specifically to softening of the articular cartilage as determined by operative observation via arthroscopy or arthrotomy. True chondromalacia reveals fractures and fissures in the cartilage that produce irregularities in the articular surfaces.[4] The exact cause of chondromalacia and patellar arthrosis is uncertain. Some degenerative changes can be expected with normal aging. Outerbridge[48] described the initial cause as the presence of an abnormal ridge on the articular surface of the femur. Fulkerson and Hungerford[17] spoke of chondromalacia at the lateral patellar facet resulting from chronic patellar tilt and increased compression forces. Medial patellar facet degeneration may result, however, from deficient synovial nutrition or increased shearing forces. Knee pain is the most common symptom associated with chondromalacia and joint arthrosis. Given that articular cartilage is aneural and avascular, the associated pain is presumed to originate from synovial irritation or bony contact in cases of significant degeneration.[5] Other symptoms associated with chondromalacia include joint grinding, instability, and stiffness. Clinical findings include patella alta, lateral tracking patella, excessive femoral or tibial torsion, internal derangement of the knee, quadriceps weakness, and excessive subtalar joint pronation.[21]

ORTHOSES

Although the specific treatment recommendations for patellofemoral dysfunctions may vary, the medical community agrees that a conservative approach may be as effective as surgery. Conservative treatment approaches include: exercise programs addressing muscular parameters of strength, flexibility, and endurance; physical agents to control pain and swelling; and external supports.[54] Various orthoses are currently being used in clinical settings for the rehabilitation of patellofemoral joint dysfunctions. This section describes the options available for orthotic intervention according to each specific pathologic condition and diagnosis. It is important to emphasize that the use of braces may help in symptom reduction, but braces are not intended to be the sole treatment for any condition. A comprehensive exercise program must be an integral part of the rehabilitation process to facilitate motor control and to optimize function.

Orthoses for Patellofemoral Pain Syndrome

The purpose of orthotic intervention in the treatment of PFPS is to help achieve and maintain optimal patellar tracking in order to prevent abnormal compression forces and degenerative changes that may result in symptoms. The most common methods of normalizing patellar tracking are through the use of knee braces, taping, and foot orthoses.

Braces

Knee braces are designed to minimize patellar compression and to guide the tracking of the patella to prevent excessive lateral shifting.[5, 13, 16, 37] Several types of patellar braces are currently available.[62] The selection of the appropriate device should be based on the individual patient's needs, the response to the appliance, and the cost.

The neoprene knee sleeve is one type of patellofemoral brace. It consists of a patellar cutout and crescent-shaped pads around the inferior and lateral aspects of the patella (Fig. 3–16A). The brace has straps designed to apply dynamic tension medially and counterbalance any lateral displacement of the patella.[49] Newer designs incorporate adjustable air chambers and detachable straps to aid in tracking of the patella, as well as in tilt, glide, and

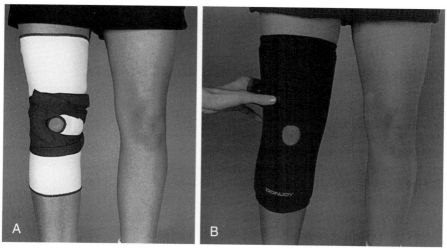

FIGURE 3–16. Braces used to control tracking of the patella. A, Palumbo Brace is a neoprene sleeve with straps to control lateral displacement of the patella. (Courtesy of DynOrthotics, Vienna, VA.) B, Air Donjoy uses a system of valves and adjustable pneumatic chambers to aid in tracking. Four detachable straps (not pictured) can be used to selectively influence patellar tilt, glide, and rotation. (Courtesy of Smith and Nephew Donjoy Inc., Carlsbad, CA.)

rotation (Fig. 3–16*B*). In addition, the brace may cause slight alterations in the tension of surrounding soft tissue to allow for optimal control of patellar tracking.[17]

Another patellofemoral brace clinically prescribed is a curved, vinyl-covered strap worn around the proximal leg just distal to the patella and fastened posteriorly with Velcro straps (Fig. 3–17). The strap is designed to support the patella distally and to alter the patellofemoral joint mechanics to facilitate accurate tracking.[32] Radiographic studies have demonstrated that the strap elevates the patella, which may relieve the compressive forces between the articular surfaces.[34]

Patellar Taping

An alternative way to optimize patellar positioning in patients with patellofemoral pain syndrome is through the use of a taping technique developed by McConnell[39] (Fig. 3–18). This taping procedure purportedly corrects the patellar orientation and controls tracking, thereby reducing pain and facilitating retraining of the VMO. To determine the need for taping, a thorough biomechanical and musculoskeletal evaluation is necessary, including evaluation of static and dynamic patellar positioning. Patients with an abnormal patellar position and typical complaints of PFPS may be candidates for patellar taping. Strips of tape are applied to hold the patella in the correct position and are worn throughout exercise and daily activities. If effective, the tape relieves or significantly reduces the patient's pain so that therapeutic exercises can be performed with the goal of developing sufficient dynamic control. As patellofemoral symptoms subside, the patient is gradually weaned from the taping procedure. (See Chap. 7 for specific taping techniques.)

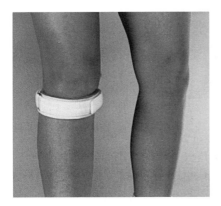

FIGURE 3–17. Infrapatellar straps can be used to elevate the patella and to facilitate optimal tracking. (Courtesy of Creative Orthotics, Ithaca, NY.)

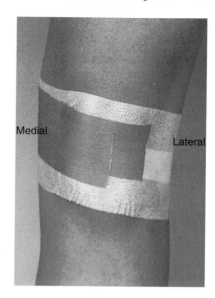

FIGURE 3–18. Specific taping techniques can be used to decrease pain, to control patellar position, and to facilitate strengthening programs in patients with patellofemoral pain syndrome.

Foot Orthoses

Another alternative in the orthotic treatment of patellofemoral pain syndrome is modification of foot alignment using foot orthoses. Research findings suggest a strong relationship between foot position and knee function.[1, 4, 9, 55, 58] As previously stated, many patients exhibit structural deviations in the foot that can adversely affect the patellofemoral joint. Most significant is excessive subtalar joint pronation, which causes a compensatory malalignment of the patellofemoral joint and an increase in compressive forces at the knee.[9, 56, 58] Treatment is recommended in patients with a forefoot or rearfoot varus or rearfoot valgus greater than 5 degrees. These alignments have been reported to cause lower-extremity symptoms related to the patellofemoral joint.[14] Orthotic devices modify the position and motion of the foot and lower extremity during stance phase of gait and reestablish normal lower-extremity position and mechanics.[4] (See Chap. 6.)

Subluxation/Dislocation

External supports for the treatment of patellar subluxation and dislocation have been used for decades. In 1939, Ober[46] suggested the use of a heel lift and a lateral patellar felt pad for the conservative treatment of these conditions. A brace consisting of a felt inverted U-pad held in place with straps was also described in 1954 as a means of securing the placement and tracking of the patella (Fig. 3–19).[47] More recently, the use of braces includes those similar to the dynamic knee supports described in the previous section, with lateral pads that prevent excessive lateral movement.[23] Foot orthoses

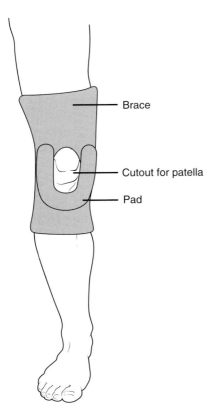

FIGURE 3-19. A brace developed in the 1950s to prevent lateral patellar tracking. The U-pad was designed to stabilize the patella.

may also be useful in improving lower-extremity alignment and in decreasing the valgus moment at the knee.[17]

Patellar Tendinitis

Various knee supports are available to help dissipate the tensile stresses on the patellar tendon and alleviate the pain.[44, 49] The braces are also believed to decrease the force of pull of the quadriceps muscle on the tibial tubercle in cases of Osgood-Schlatter disease.[57] These include elastic sleeves and infrapatellar straps such as the Palumbo Brace and Cho-Pat Strap. Foot orthoses may also be used to dampen the impact of initial contact on the extensor mechanism.[57] Additionally, McConnell[40] has proposed the use of tape in creating a relief around the patellar tendon so forces are "unloaded" and the tendon is allowed to heal (Fig. 3–20).

EFFECTIVENESS OF CLINICAL TRIALS

Although orthoses are frequently included as part of a comprehensive treatment plan, there is little empirical research supporting the effectiveness of

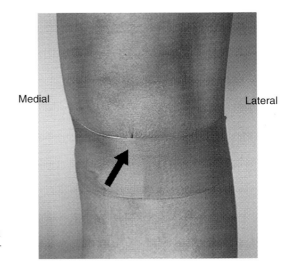

FIGURE 3-20. Tape can be applied to create a "relief" around a tendon and to reduce stress, thereby allowing time for healing. Note that the skin appears pinched *(arrow)* together overlying the patellar tendon.

braces or the various methods of orthotic intervention for treatment of patellofemoral joint dysfunction. In a study of 100 athletes with a clinical diagnosis of chondromalacia patellae, DeHaven et al[10] found an 82% success rate (subjects were able to resume activities with no pain) following participation in a conservative management program. This regimen consisted of progressive strengthening exercises for the quadriceps and hamstrings, a running program, and a maintenance program including knee braces and foot orthoses as indicated. In a similar study of conservative management of 370 patients with PFPS, Malek and Mangine[36] reported satisfactory results in 77% of the population. These authors used a four-stage treatment approach that included management of acute symptoms, exercises to increase the strength and flexibility of the lower extremity, eccentric and endurance training, and return to activity with the use of external supports as needed. In 145 patients with patellar subluxation, Henry and Crosland[24] demonstrated a 76% success rate with a program of resisted straight leg raises, hip abduction, hip flexion, and the use of an elastic knee bandage with a lateral felt pad during running or sports. Subjective data revealed that 64% of those patients who improved felt that the brace was helpful.

In an early study that evaluated the effectiveness of an infrapatellar strap, Levine and Splain[34] examined 57 patients with patellofemoral pain. Subjects were instructed to wear the strap only during periods of activity, and no mention was made of an exercise program. Seventy-seven percent of the patients reported sufficient pain relief to allow them to resume normal activity. Doppler flow studies also revealed no impedance of venous circulation with the use of the strap. Conflicting results were found by Villar[60] in a study of 37 subjects who had PFPS. Following 2 weeks of wearing an infrapatellar brace during normal activity, only 22% reported complete relief of symptoms, 24% reported partial relief, and 54% indicated no change in symptoms. All the subjects who reported relief of symptoms after the initial two weeks of wearing the strap continued to report good results in a 1-year follow-up study.

Several studies have examined the effectiveness of the patellar brace. In 62 patients with a diagnosis of patellar subluxation, severe chondromalacia, or Osgood-Schlatter disease, Palumbo[49] found that 93% reported a significant reduction in symptoms while wearing the Palumbo Brace. The patients were able to perform activities with the brace that they previously were unable to do, including pivoting, running, stair climbing, and long-distance walking. Forty-eight percent of the patients with recurrent patellar subluxation reported that they wore the brace only during athletic activities. In another study, Moller and Krebs[41] compared two groups of patients with similar complaints of anterior knee pain. The patients were divided into a control (n = 17) group and an experimental (n = 17) group. Both groups performed quadriceps strengthening exercises for a 6-week period. The experimental group also wore a hinged knee brace that allowed range of motion from 0 to 30 degrees. The authors reported an 82% success rate as determined by improvement in symptoms and/or elimination of pain in those subjects who wore the brace, compared to 44% improvement in the exercise-only group. Additionally, no subjects demonstrated evidence of muscle atrophy as determined by circumferential measurements of the thigh. These findings support the use of an orthotic device in combination with an exercise program in the conservative treatment of patellofemoral dysfunction.

In addition to improving subjective complaints and functional ability, bracing facilitates motor strength and control. In a study of 24 patients with anterior knee pain, Lysholm et al[35] assessed the effect of an elastic sleeve with a patellar cutout and lateral pad on isokinetic concentric quadriceps strength. Eighty-eight percent of the subjects produced greater torque output when wearing the brace. The author suggested that control of patellar tracking enhances torque output but recommended further investigation to examine braces with and without lateral padding. The study also revealed that patients under the age of 30 responded better to the brace than did older patients, possibly because the source of patellar pain in older people may be due to actual degenerative changes in the joint surfaces rather than to maltracking.

Patellar taping has become a common method of treating patellofemoral dysfunction, although the mechanism of its effectiveness remains unknown. In a study of 35 patients with PFPS, McConnell[39] reported decreased or no pain in 92% of the patients after eight treatments of taping and a progressive strengthening program. At a 6-month follow-up, 40% of these patients remained pain-free and compliant with the exercise program. The study also reported an increase in VMO electromyographic activity during isometric quadriceps contraction with taping. The author concluded that taping reduces pain and facilitates accurate tracking to enable the quadriceps to function as a dynamic stabilizer of the patella. Gerrard[18] obtained similar results in a study of 116 patients treated with the McConnell regimen of tape and exercise. Ninety percent of patients reported pain relief after seven treatment sessions, and a follow-up questionnaire 12 months later revealed that results were maintained. In 28% of the subjects, symptoms returned if the exercises were stopped, indicating the importance of maintaining an exercise program.

Although the effectiveness of taping appears comparable to that of other orthotic interventions, the mechanism by which it is effective remains unclear. McConnell[39] proposed that correction of patellar alignment decreases pain and allows for optimal training and recruitment of the VMO. Hilyard et al[25] compared the torque output and electromyographic activity in 14 patients with patellofemoral pain using both the McConnell taping technique and a placebo taping. No significant differences in torque output or electromyographic activity were found between the two groups, suggesting that the effects of taping may be related to cutaneous sensory input or to psychological factors. The results of a study by Bockrath et al[3] examining the effect of tape on patellar position and pain support the previous conclusions. Using radiography, the authors observed no change in the position of the patella with taping, but pain complaints decreased significantly. The authors hypothesized that pain reduction in the absence of patellar position changes may be related to sensory input. One limitation of this study, however, was that the radiographs were taken at a static position of 45 degrees of knee flexion, whereas pain was assessed through a functional movement. Further studies are needed to examine the effect of taping on the patellar position at different knee joint angles and throughout dynamic movement.

In 1992, Conway et al[7] compared the effects of the Palumbo Brace and McConnell taping on torque output at 60 degrees per second and pain perception in 30 patients with anterior knee pain. When compared to the control trial (no external support), both taping and the brace conditions resulted in a significantly increased torque output of the quadriceps. Both concentric and eccentric torque output increased with taping whereas only eccentric torque output increased with the brace. Perceived pain was lower with both orthotic interventions, although the reduced pain did not correlate with the observed changes in torque production. The authors proposed that other factors may have affected the results, including biomechanical advantages, neurologic factors due to tactile and proprioceptive input, and psychological factors.

As previously discussed, the position of the foot affects the function of the knee. The use of shoe orthoses to correct foot alignment can therefore be assumed to affect dysfunctions of the patellofemoral joint. In a survey of 146 runners treated for running-related injuries, the most prevalent complaint (40%) was knee pain.[12] Of these respondents, 100% obtained complete relief of symptoms with orthotic intervention. Eng and Pierrynowski[14] studied 20 female adolescents with PFPS. The experimental group performed the same exercises as the control group, but the subjects were also given soft foot orthoses. Patients were followed for 8 weeks, and pain perceptions were collected using a visual analog scale. Although both groups reported a decrease in pain, a significantly greater decrease in knee pain was found in those subjects who wore orthoses. This finding may be related to decreased tibial internal rotation movement resulting from controlled pronation.[43] The effect of foot orthoses on the Q angle and associated patellofemoral joint has also been assessed using the weight-bearing Q angle measurement. D'Amico and Rubin[9] showed that the use of a foot orthosis decreased the Q angle measurements in 85.7% of patients (n = 21) with patellofemoral joint pain. This decreased Q angle may alter the forces acting on the patellofemoral joint and may decrease the tendency for lateral displacement of the patella.

SUMMARY

Although the most effective treatment approach to patellofemoral dysfunctions is still under discussion, the overwhelming consensus is that a conservative approach is preferred. The use of knee braces, taping, or foot orthoses can be an important component of a comprehensive program of strengthening and flexibility exercises designed to achieve dynamic control and balance at the patellofemoral joint. Further studies are needed to explore mechanisms for orthotic effectiveness in patients with PFPS, and to compare orthotic interventions in various clinical settings.

REFERENCES

1. Bates BT, Osternig LR, Mason B, James LS: Foot orthotic devices to modify selected aspects of lower extremity mechanics. Am J Sports Med 7:338–342, 1979.
2. Bennett GB, Stauber WT: Evaluation and treatment of anterior knee pain using eccentric exercise. Med Sci Sports Exerc 18:526–530, 1986.
3. Bockrath K, Wooden C, Worrell T, et al: Effects of patella taping on patella position and perceived pain. Med Sci Sports Exerc 25:989–992, 1993.
4. Buchbinder MR, Napora NJ, Biggs EW: The relationship of abnormal pronation to chondromalacia of the patella in distance runners. J Am Podiatr Med Assoc 69:159–162, 1979.
5. Calliet R: Knee Pain and Disability, 3rd ed, Philadelphia, F.A. Davis Co., 1992, pp 103–104.
6. Carson WG: Diagnosis of extensor mechanism disorders. Clin Sports Med 4:231–246, 1985.
7. Conway A, Malone TR, Conway P: Patellar alignment/tracking alteration: Effect on force output and perceived pain. Isokinet Exerc Sci 2:9–17, 1992.
8. Curwin S, Standish WD: Tendinitis: Its Etiology and Treatment, Lexington, Collamore Press, 1984.
9. D'Amico JC, Rubin M: The influence of foot orthoses on quadriceps angle. J Am Podiatr Med Assoc 76:337–340, 1986.
10. DeHaven KE, Dolan WA, Mayer PJ: Chondromalacia patellae in athletes: Clinical presentation and conservative management. Am J Sports Med 7:5–11, 1979.

11. Dugdale TW, Barnett PR: Historical background: Patellofemoral pain in young people. Orthop Clin North Am 17:211–219, 1986.
12. Eggold JF: Orthotics in the prevention of runners' overuse injuries. Physician Sportsmed 9:125–131, 1981.
13. Eisele SA: A precise approach to anterior knee pain. Phys Sports Med 19:126–139, 1991.
14. Eng JJ, Pierrynowski MR: Evaluation of soft foot orthotics in the treatment of patellofemoral pain syndrome. Phys Ther 73:62–68, 1993.
15. Ericson MO, Nisell R: Patellofemoral joint forces during cycling. Phys Ther 67:1365–1369, 1987.
16. Fisher RL: Conservative treatment of patellofemoral pain. Orthop Clin North Am 17:269–272, 1986.
17. Fulkerson JP, Hungerford DS: Disorders of the Patellofemoral Joint, 2nd ed, Baltimore, Williams & Wilkins, 1990, pp 3, 26, 38, 98–99, 176–220.
18. Gerrard B: The patellofemoral pain syndrome: A clinical trial of the McConnell programme. Aust J Physiother 35:71–80, 1989.
19. Goodfellow JW, Hungerford DS, Zindell M: Patellofemoral joint mechanics and pathology. J Bone Joint Surg (Br) 58:287–299, 1976.
20. Grana WA, Kriegshauser LA: Scientific basis of extensor mechanism disorders. Clin Sports Med 4:247–257, 1985.
21. Greenfield BH: Rehabilitation of the Knee: A Problem-Solving Approach, Philadelphia, F.A. Davis Co., 1993.
22. Gruber MA: The conservative treatment of chondromalacia patellae. Orthop Clin North Am 10:105–115, 1979.
23. Henry JH: Conservative treatment of patellofemoral subluxation. Orthop Clin North Am 8:261–278, 1989.
24. Henry JH, Crosland JW: Conservative treatment of patellofemoral subluxation. Am J Sports Med 7:12–14, 1979.
25. Hilyard A, Moore C, Pope J: McConnell taping: Does it really work? (abstract) Aust J Physiother 35:194, 1989.
26. Huberti HH, Hayes WC: Patellofemoral contact pressure. J Bone Joint Surg (A) 66:715–724, 1984.
27. Hughston JC: Patellar subluxation: A recent history. Clin Sports Med 8:153–162, 1989.
28. Hungerford DS, Barry M: Biomechanics of the patellofemoral joint. Clin Orthop 144:9–15, 1979.
29. Insall J: Chondromalacia patellae: Patellar malalignment syndrome. Orthop Clin North Am 10:117–125, 1979.
30. James SL, Bates BT, Osternig LR: Injuries to runners. Am J Sports Med 6:40–50, 1978.
31. Kramer PG: Patella malalignment syndrome: Rationale to reduce excessive lateral pressure. J Orthop Sports Phys Ther 8:301–309, 1986.
32. Levine J: A new brace for chondromalacia patella and kindred conditions. Am J Sports Med 6:137–140, 1978.
33. Levine J: Chondromalacia patellae. Physician Sportsmed 7:41–49, 1979.
34. Levine J, Splain S: Use of the infrapatellar strap in the treatment of patellofemoral pain. Clin Orthop Rel Res 139:179–181, 1979.
35. Lysholm J, Nordin M, Ekstrand J, Gillquist J: The effect of a patella brace on performance in knee extension strength test in patients with patellar pain. Am J Sports Med 12:110–112, 1984.
36. Malek M, Mangine R: Patellofemoral pain syndromes: A comprehensive and conservative approach. J Orthop Sports Phys Ther 2:108–116, 1981.
37. Malone T, Blackburn TA, Wallace LA: Knee rehabilitation. Phys Ther 60:1602–1610, 1980.
38. Martens M, Wourters P, Burssens A, et al: Patellar tendinitis: Pathology and results of treatment. Acta Orthop Scand 53:445–450, 1982.
39. McConnell J: The management of chondromalacia patellae: A long-term solution. Aust J Physiother 32:215–223, 1986.
40. McConnell J: McConnell Patellofemoral Treatment Plan (from course notes). 1991, p 59.
41. Moller BN, Krebs B: Dynamic knee brace in the treatment of patellofemoral disorders. Arch Orthop Trauma Surg 104:377–379, 1986.
42. Moss RI, DeVita P, Dawson ML: A biomechanical analysis of patellofemoral stress syndrome. J Athletic Training 27:64–69, 1992.
43. Nawoczenski DA, Cook TM, Saltzman CL: The effect of foot orthotics on three-dimensional

kinematics of the leg and rearfoot during running. J Orthop Sports Phys Ther 21:317–327, 1995.
44. Nichols CE: Patellar tendon injuries. Clin Sports Med 11:807–812, 1992.
45. Norkin CC, Levangie PK: Joint Structure and Function: A Comprehensive Analysis, 2nd ed, Philadelphia, F.A. Davis Co., 1992.
46. Ober FR: Recurrent dislocation of the patella. Am J Surg 43:497–500, 1939.
47. Orr HW: A review of the surgical treatment of congenital dislocation, recurrent dislocation, or slipping patella. Clin Orthop 3:3–7, 1954.
48. Outerbridge RE: The etiology of chondromalacia patellae. J Bone Joint Surg (Br) 43:752–757, 1961.
49. Palumbo PM: Dynamic patellar brace: A new orthosis in the management of patellofemoral disorders. Am J Sports Med 9:45–49, 1981.
50. Paulos L, Rusche K, Johnson C, et al: Patellar malalignment: A treatment rationale. Phys Ther 60:1624–1632, 1980.
51. Ramig D, Shadle J, Watkins CA, et al: The foot and sports medicine—biomechanical foot faults as related to chondromalacia patellae. J Orthop Sports Phys Ther 2:48–53, 1980.
52. Roels J, Martens M, Mulier JC, et al: Patellar tendinitis. Am J Sports Med 6:362–368, 1978.
53. Shellock FG, Mink JH, Deutsch A, et al: Kinematic magnetic resonance imaging for evaluation of patellar tracking. Physician Sportsmed 17:99–108, 1989.
54. Shelton GL, Thigpen LK: Rehabilitation of patellofemoral dysfunction: A review of literature. J Orthop Sports Phys Ther 14:243–249, 1991.
55. Steadman JR: Non-operative measures for patellofemoral problems. Am J Sports Med 7:374–375, 1979.
56. Tauton JE, Clement DB, Smart GW, et al: Non-surgical management of overuse knee injures in runners. Can J Sport Sci 12:11–18, 1987.
57. Thabit G, Micheli LJ: Patellofemoral pain in the pediatric patient. Orthop Clin North Am 23:567–585, 1992.
58. Tiberio D: The effect of excessive subtalar joint pronation on patellofemoral mechanics: A theoretical model. J Orthop Sports Phys Ther 9:160–165, 1987.
59. Tria AJ, Palumbo RC, Alicea JA: Conservative care for patellofemoral pain. Orthop Clin North Am 23:545–554, 1992.
60. Villar RN: Patellofemoral pain and the infrapatellar brace: A military view. Am J Sports Med 13:313–315, 1985.
61. Wiberg B: Roentgenographic and anatomical studies of the femoropatellar joint, with special reference to chondromalacia patellae. Acta Orthop Scand 12:319, 1941.
62. Willis J: The knee brace source list. Biomechanics 11:33–40, 1995.
63. Woodall W, Welsh J: A biomechanical basis for rehabilitation programs involving the patellofemoral joint. J Orthop Sports Phys Ther 11:535–541, 1990.

CHAPTER 4

Orthoses for the Knee: The Tibiofemoral Joint

TJ ANTICH

The knee joint is frequently subjected to great amounts of force that can be transferred to the surrounding ligaments and static soft tissue restraints. When the weight-bearing limb is in a position in which external forces exceed the strength of the knee's support structures, an injury is likely to occur. Following an injury to the knee, brace prescription is often an integral part of the rehabilitation process.

LIGAMENTOUS ANATOMY

The anterior cruciate ligament (ACL) and posterior cruciate ligament (PCL), located centrally and posteriorly in the knee joint, are responsible for limiting excessive movement of the tibia in their respective directions (Fig. 4–1). Through cadaver dissection studies, Butler et al[6] demonstrated that the human ACL provides 95% of the passive restraint of forward movement of the tibia, and the PCL provides 86% of the passive restraint of posterior translation of the leg on the thigh.

France and Paulos[10] demonstrated that the medial collateral ligament (MCL) provides 80% of the restraint to a valgus load, with the balance of resistance split between the ACL and PCL. As the magnitude of an imposed valgus force increases, the stress may be transmitted from the MCL to the cruciate ligaments. As a result, the likelihood of subsequent injury to the cruciate ligaments is increased. At the moment of simultaneous failure of all three ligaments, the knee joint opens approximately 57 mm.

PATHOMECHANICS OF ACL INJURY

In athletic competition, a twisting injury to a planted, weight-bearing lower extremity is the most common mechanism of injury resulting in acute ACL tear. With the knee slightly flexed and the foot fixed on the ground, internal rotation of the femur combined with a valgus stress at the knee can stress the ligament beyond the point of ultimate failure. In direct or nondirect mechanisms of injury, the athlete may hear or feel a "pop" resulting from the speed at which the ligament exceeds its tensile potential.

At the instant of ligament disruption, the buckling of the loaded knee frequently results in the athlete's falling to the ground. The individual is usually unable to continue the sporting activity and usually requires assistance to the sidelines. Owing to the abundant vascular supply to the ACL, bleeding occurs within the capsule of the knee joint, resulting in an immediate hemarthrosis.

Orthopaedic evaluation of an acute ACL tear encompasses a combination of clinical straight-plane and rotational tests to determine both static and dynamic laxity. Decisions regarding conservative versus surgical management of an ACL-deficient knee are based on the age and activity level of the patient, degree of functional instability, and presence or absence of associated injuries.

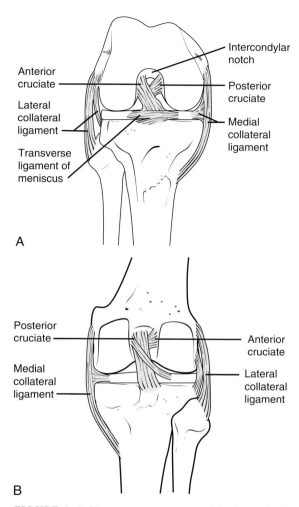

FIGURE 4-1. Ligamentous structures of the knee. A, Anterior view. B, Posterior view.

Following a course of rehabilitation, functional bracing is usually recommended for return to high-stress sports that involve stop-and-go running, cutting, twisting, and pivoting maneuvers. The primary objective of functional bracing in these patients is to decrease knee hyperextension as well as to decrease excessive anterior tibial translation or tibial rotation.

ORTHOSES

Knee Immobilizers

Plaster casts, the primary means of immobilization in past years, have been replaced by Velcro immobilizers. This lighter, less expensive means of immobilization, which is less time-consuming for the physician to apply, offers the patient the added benefit of increased comfort by allowing daily showering. Optimal soft tissue healing based on principles of ligament biomechanics as well as the specific mechanism of injury determine whether the knee is immobilized in a position of full extension or in some degree of knee flexion.

Prophylactic Knee Braces

The 1984 Knee Brace Seminar Report of the American Academy of Orthopaedic Surgeons defines prophylactic knee braces as "those designed to prevent or reduce the severity of knee injuries."[9] The characteristics of an ideal prophylactic brace include the following[9, 16]:

- supplementing the stiffness of the knee against injury-producing loads from both contact and noncontact stresses
- not interfering with normal function
- not increasing risk factors elsewhere in the lower extremity
- being adaptable to various anatomic shapes and sizes
- not being harmful to other players
- being cost-effective and durable
- having documented efficacy in preventing injuries

Prophylactic braces are generally worn by athletes with normal knee structure in an attempt to protect the knee during sports activities. These braces were originally marketed for use by offensive and defensive football linemen to minimize an injury should one lineman fall onto the lateral side of the knee of another lineman. Prophylactic braces were also recommended for other position players, such as linebackers and tight ends, who were thought to be at a higher-than-normal risk for knee ligament injuries.[24]

The first-generation prophylactic knee braces were constructed primarily of a lateral bar with either a single- or a dual-axis hinge, along with range-of-motion stops that prevented hyperextension of the athlete's knee. Some models of these braces were affixed to the lateral thigh and leg by straps or tape, whereas other models made with plastic cuffs and polycentric hinges could be custom-molded to the player's leg.[9] Specific models of prophylactic braces are described in this section.

McDAVID KNEE GUARD. The McDavid Knee Guard (McDavid Knee Guard, Inc., Clarendon Hills, IL) originally entered the market around 1967 as a rehabilitative brace. As early as 1969, this brace was also found suitable for use as a prophylactic brace designed to prevent medial and lateral stress injuries. The McDavid Knee Guard is composed of a single lateral bar with a single-axis hinge with hyperextension stops, which is affixed to the limb with tape or elastic wraps.

ANDERSON KNEE STABLER. The Anderson Knee Stabler (Omni Scientific, Inc., Lafayette, IL) is a single lateral steel support secured to the thigh and leg with tape. This off-the-shelf brace contains a dual-axis hinge with hyperextension stops and a polypropylene lateral cuff. Because of its direct contact with the skin, minor problems with skin irritation have been reported with this brace.[1]

Effectiveness in Clinical Trials

Several studies have attempted to provide epidemiologic data correlating the decreased likelihood of major ligamentous injury with the use of prophylactic braces in football players. To date, clinical investigations have been unable to consistently demonstrate the efficacy of these braces.

Some clinical studies performed in the mid-1980s demonstrated a reduction in the frequency of MCL injuries in athletes wearing single lateral upright braces.[12, 21] Conversely, Rovere et al[19] and Teitz et al[23] noted an increased rate of injury when prophylactic braces were worn as well as a failure of the brace to protect either the ACL or the MCL. Paulos and associates[16] reported consistent MCL disruption in braced and unbraced cadaveric knees following application of valgus forces. Additionally, other possible harmful effects included preloading of the MCL, shifting of the center axis, early joint line contact, and brace slippage.[17] A study by Hewson et al[13] revealed no differences in football injury rates for players with braced versus unbraced knees. Sitler et al[20] reported a reduction in the frequency, but not in the severity, of MCL injuries in braced defensive players.

France et al[11] studied the biomechanics of lateral knee bracing. They concluded that the greatest protection to the MCL was provided by stiffer braces in which the lateral hinge was not in close contact with the knee and in which applied forces allowed deformation of the metal.

The effectiveness of prophylactic bracing remains unclear. Footwear characteristics, various playing surfaces, and nonstandardized terminology and methodology of clinical studies all have contributed to the conflicting viewpoints regarding the efficacy of prophylactic knee bracing. What constitutes a reportable injury is frequently discussed in the literature. The most widely accepted definition of a reportable injury is an "acute trauma to ligaments that results in an athlete's inability to participate in football one day after the injury."[20]

Rehabilitative Braces

Approximately 15 years ago, it was accepted practice for an individual undergoing ACL reconstruction to be immobilized in 45 degrees of flexion in a long leg cast. It then became apparent, through the work of Salter in Canada and Noyes in the United States, that early controlled motion was actually beneficial in producing a stronger ligament during the early rehabilitation phase. This finding led to the concept of "cast-bracing" in which the patient was allowed to gradually increase the arc of knee motion as determined by the surgeon. It was not long until the transition was made to prefabricated off-the-shelf braces, which greatly reduced the physician's time requirement and could easily be applied in the recovery room following surgery.

Rehabilitative braces are prescribed in the conservative treatment and postoperative management of knee ligament injuries. The 1984 Knee Braces Seminar Report defines rehabilitative braces as those "which are designed to allow protected motion of injured knees or knees that have been treated operatively."[9] Although these braces can allow full knee range of motion, adjustable stops are commonly incorporated to maintain the knee in a limited protective range of motion.[24] The 1984 Knee Brace Seminar Report[9] lists the desirable features of rehabilitation braces as follows:

- providing accurate control of knee motions so that excessive loads on healing tissues are avoided
- remaining in position without slippage
- adapting to various leg sizes and shapes and being available as off-the-shelf items
- adapting for edema and atrophy
- being comfortable for the user
- being easily applied and removed
- allowing the brace to be locked at a given joint angle
- being durable and economical

Rehabilitative braces offer the orthopaedic surgeon and physical therapist the ability to unlock the brace for early range-of-motion activities. Additionally, the patient can either unlock the brace for sitting activities requiring flexion or lock the brace in full extension, thereby preventing the likelihood of scar tissue formation in the intracondylar notch and subsequent knee flexion contracture. If collateral ligament surgery is performed in conjunction with cruciate ligament reconstruction, the surgeon may choose to lock the brace in a position of slight flexion to minimize stress on that structure during the initial healing phase.

TWO-PHASE/BREAKDOWN VARIETY. Several brace companies have produced two-phase/breakdown braces that the patient can wear through much of the postoperative rehabilitation phases of treatment. This type of brace can be fit immediately after surgery and can continue to be worn all through the rehabilitation process. Two-phase/breakdown orthoses are a cost-effective means of providing the appropriate amount of protection for the knee throughout the postoperative regimen.

Most rehabilitation braces are off-the-shelf models that are easily applied. They can be adjusted as the patient's thigh and calf girth changes during rehabilitation. Additionally, bracing, as opposed to postoperative casting, tends to be much cooler for the patient, especially during the summer months, and allows early aquatic therapy intervention once the incision is fully healed.

Formerly, most patients were advised to wear the rehabilitation brace during physical therapy to protect the knee and to help minimize anterior drawing of the tibia during isolated quadriceps open-kinetic chain exercise. Recently, many orthopaedic surgeons have opted to allow patients to exercise without wearing any rehabilitation brace, reserving the use of a brace for subsequent return to cutting and twisting activities.

DONJOY SYSTEM 2 REHABILITATIVE BRACE. The DonJoy System 2 Rehabilitative Brace (Smith & Nephew DonJoy, Inc., Carlsbad, CA) is constructed of polycentric hinges that contain variable flexion and extension stops. Foam underwraps are worn under the thigh and calf, and an additional antiedema wrap can be applied to compress excessive joint swelling. This brace is available off-the-shelf and can be broken down to a shorter version as the patient improves.

DONJOY ELS REHABILITATIVE BRACE. The DonJoy ELS Rehabilitative Brace is a newer version of a two-phase brace. Its highlights include the ability to lock the brace in full knee extension or unlock the brace to allow full movement during therapy (Fig. 4–2). This feature makes this brace ideal for patients recovering from fractures because it can support the limb in extension during weight bearing while allowing the knee to flex when the patient is sitting. The medial and lateral metal supports are perforated at both the femoral and the tibial ends to allow a medical professional to manually shorten the brace in minutes.

BLEDSOE BRACE. The Bledsoe Brace (Bledsoe Brace Systems, Grand Prairie, TX) features double upright hinge bars that have a partial circumference lightweight shell bilaterally. Further, a removable posterior lower-limb shell provides a broader area of support. The simple hinge joint allows control of range of motion for either strict immobilization or limited arcs. The brace requires a small Allen wrench for adjustment.

DONJOY IROM. The DonJoy IROM Brace (Fig. 4–3) features double upright aluminum alloy hinge bars that are prescored to convert to a short brace version for interim rehabilitation brace requirements. The simple hinge joint locks to provide strict immobilization or opens to controlled arcs of motion from 0 to 80 degrees of extension and 0 to 120 degrees of flexion (in 10-degree increments). The nonelastic Velcro straps provide control and circumferential compression.

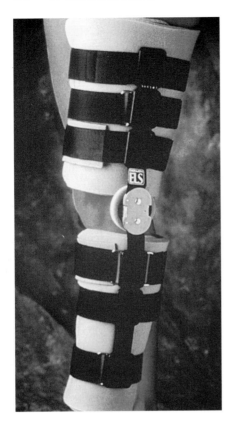

FIGURE 4-2. DonJoy ELS Rehabilitative Brace. (Courtesy of Smith & Nephew DonJoy, Inc., Carlsbad, CA.)

Effectiveness in Clinical Trials

Stevenson et al[22] and Cawley et al[7] reported that patients wearing rehabilitative braces were able to achieve 15 to 20 degrees of extension more than the brace allowed. Clinicians are advised not to place too much emphasis on the readings of the brace dials as an accurate representation of the actual angle of the knee flexion and extension.

Functional ACL Knee Braces

Functional knee braces are those worn by individuals who have returned to activity. They are "designed to provide increased stability for an unstable knee."[9] Use of this type of orthosis was popularized in the late 1960s and early 1970s in extending Joe Namath's football career following multiple ligament operations on both knees. Necessary requirements for functional stability include the following:

• satisfactory primary and secondary ligament restraints

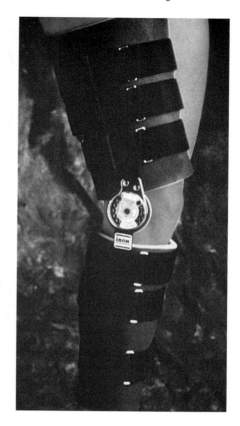

FIGURE 4–3. DonJoy IROM Brace. (Courtesy of Smith & Nephew DonJoy, Inc., Carlsbad, CA.)

- static, compressive joint forces along with dynamic forces resulting from muscle contraction
- proprioceptive and neuromuscular input to integrate the necessary co-contraction of agonist and antagonistic muscles

When prescribing a functional brace for return to sports or other vigorous activities, the health care professional should allow the patient to have considerable input regarding fit, comfort, and appearance.

HINGE, POST, AND STRAP

LENOX HILL BRACE. The Lenox Hill Brace (3M Health Care, Long Island City, NY), originally designed in 1969, is a double upright, single-hinge brace held in place with proximal and distal straps (Fig. 4–4). A medial fulcrum pad assists in positioning the brace against the distal femur, and a second lateral condyle pad is available for patients as needed. The derotation straps are narrow for increased comfort, and the absence of metal in the patellar region makes the brace safer for opponents in contact sports.

The metal thigh and tibial sections make adjustments easier by allowing

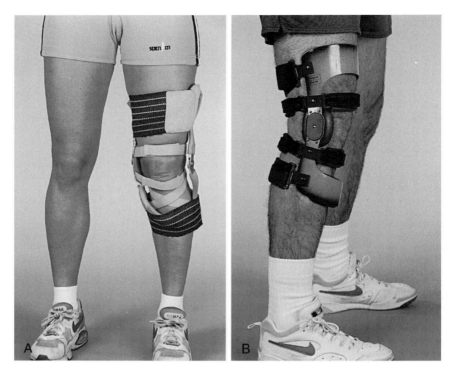

FIGURE 4-4. *A*, Lenox Hill Brace. *B*, Lenox Hill Precision Fit Brace.

the orthotist to bend and to reshape both the proximal and the distal pieces. It is the only brace with a dial lock for adjusting range of motion and is available in three different weights: standard, lightweight, and the newest weight of between 18 and 23 ounces (the Spectralight).

This custom brace can be upgraded with features such as a protective outer sports sleeve that is especially helpful for wrestlers, a limited motion attachment, and a knee undersleeve.

OMNI AVANT GARDE. The OMNI Avant Garde (OMNI Scientific, Inc., Layfayette, IL), a carbon-composite hinge, post, and strap brace, is easily adjustable for changing thigh and calf circumference during rehabilitation via the patented X-CELL thigh restraint strap system (Fig. 4–5). A pretibial buttress is built into the proximal anterior tibial strap to further control anterior tibial migration. A heat gun can be used to remold the shell. Although primarily a functional knee orthosis, a gravity-extension locking system (GELS) and a variable flexion overhinge (VFO) allow controlled range of motion if needed early in the postoperative rehabilitation stages.

The OMNI TS-7, an earlier and similarly priced version of the Avant Garde, is heavier and bulkier with more straps.

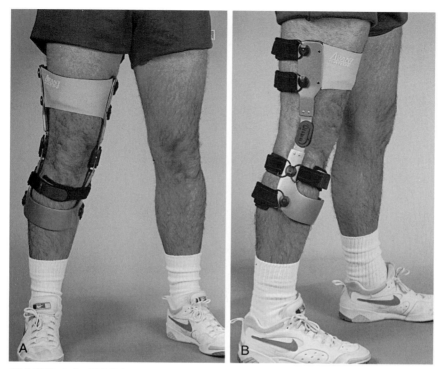

FIGURE 4–5. OMNI Avant Garde Brace. *A,* Anterior view. *B,* Lateral view.

DONJOY GOLDPOINT. The DonJoy GoldPoint Brace (Smith & Nephew DonJoy, Inc., Carlsbad, CA) is an off-the-shelf four-point brace that consists of a rigid medial and lateral superstructure connecting semicircular anterior and posterior thigh pieces to a polyaxial hinge (Fig. 4–6). This hinge possesses adjustable flexion and extension stops. Velcro thigh and calf straps connect directly to the superstructure, and two additional overstraps course outside the brace at the thigh and calf levels. Comfortable chamois thigh and calf pads render an undersleeve unnecessary. Condylar pads of various sizes accommodate many girths, and a pretibial strap may be tightened to provide greater resistance to anterior tibial translation.

HINGE, POST, AND SHELL

CTi BRACE. The CTi Brace (Innovation Sports, Irvine, CA) is a custom-fit brace made of a carbon-titanium alloy weighing 15 to 18 ounces. The CTi is constructed from a rigid anterior shell connected to a polyaxial hinge. Adjustable extension blocks are incorporated, and the Velcro strapping system is attached directly to the superstructure (Fig. 4–7). Rubber padding softens the condyle pads, thereby allowing firm contact with the medial and lateral skin areas.

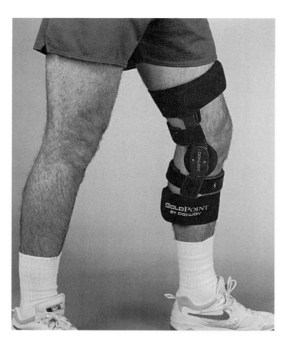

FIGURE 4–6. DonJoy GoldPoint Brace.

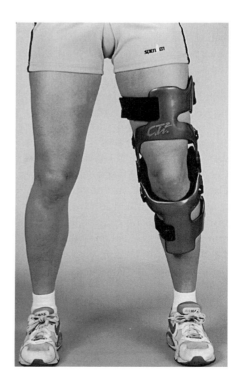

FIGURE 4–7. CTi Brace.

The CTi, which provides more lateral than medial support, tends to slip down the leg. Using only Velcro straps, it may not hug the knee as tightly as other brands do. Increased proximal tibial pressure must be monitored. The ability of this brace to withstand the rigors and impact of American football has been questioned. The CTi comes in three different weights: standard, pro-sport, and super-light. This brace can be upgraded to include a ski boot attachment, a patellar cup, or an ACL cable system to limit knee joint range of motion.

CAN-AM BRACE. The Can-Am Brace, developed in Ottawa, Ontario, Canada, and modified in Boston, Massachusetts, incorporates a posterior strap to prevent knee hyperextension. The double-upright brace extends 9 inches on both sides of the knee joint and is built with either 3/16-inch aluminum or 5/8-inch stainless steel. Polycentric hinges join the proximal and distal lateral uprights in this brace.

The Pro-Am Brace is a modification of the Can-Am brace.

TOWNSEND BRACE. The Townsend Brace (Townsend Design, Bakersfield, CA) is composed of femoral and tibial shells fabricated from carbon fiber and epoxy. The anterior tibial shell encircles approximately 65% of the circumference of the limb, thereby providing a posterior pressure to protect the ACL as the knee moves into full extension. The femoral and tibial shells are joined by a hinge that allows for a roll and glide mechanism that mimics the movement patterns of the human knee (Fig. 4–8). The manufacturer reports a 9-mm posterior tibial movement during the first 25 degrees of knee flexion. The hinge allows for adjustable flexion and extension stops. This custom-made brace is fabricated from a cast of the individual's injured lower extremity. The cast is shipped to California in a 1- to 2-day turnaround. The neoprene lining eliminates the need to wear an undersleeve.

DONJOY DEFIANCE. The DonJoy Defiance (Smith & Nephew DonJoy, Inc., Carlsbad, CA) is one of the easiest off-the-shelf functional braces to apply. It is also comfortably light, weighing 18 ounces. Manufactured around a geared polycentric hinge, the Defiance possesses the ability to allow full knee extension or to limit movement to a more neutral position of 10, 20, 30, or 40 degrees of flexion. Knee flexion can be limited by inserting shims of different sizes in the hinge area to block motion to 45, 60, 75, or 90 degrees (Fig. 4–9).

The anterior thigh frame and posterior calf frame are held in place by elasticized straps. Medial and lateral condyle pads help secure the carbon-composite frame in a proper anatomic alignment. The thigh and leg sections are available in shorter lengths for individuals with smaller inseams.

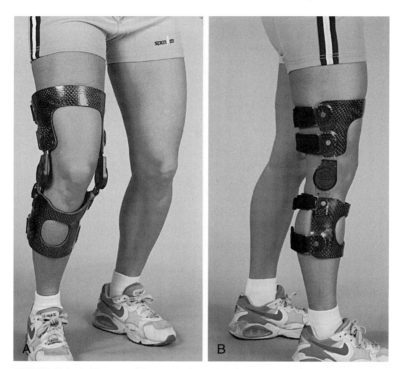

FIGURE 4-8. Townsend Brace. A, Anterior view. B, Lateral view.

DONJOY CE2000. The DonJoy CE2000 (Smith & Nephew DonJoy, Inc., Carlsbad, CA) is a heavy-duty brace recommended for those who play high-contact sports (Fig. 4–10). Because some athletes dislike the heavier weight of this brace, it is best suited for large football players.

Effectiveness in Clinical Trials

Athletes frequently question if wearing a functional knee brace will diminish performance levels. Houston and Goemans[14] documented a 30% decrease in knee strength measured isokinetically, but only at the high test speed of 300 degrees per second. Zetterlund et al[25] noted a 4.58% increase in oxygen consumption and a 5.1% increase in heart rate during horizontal treadmill running at 6 mph while subjects were wearing a functional brace on one knee. Branch et al[5] reported a 15% and 16% decrease in quadriceps and medial hamstring EMG activity, respectively, during the stance phase of straight cutting using the Lenox Hill Brace and the CTi Brace.

Bassett and Fleming[2] reported improved knee stability during testing with a brace, although 70% of subjects still demonstrated intermittent functional instability while using the brace for activity.

Bassett and Fleming[2] also studied the effect of the Lenox Hill Brace on

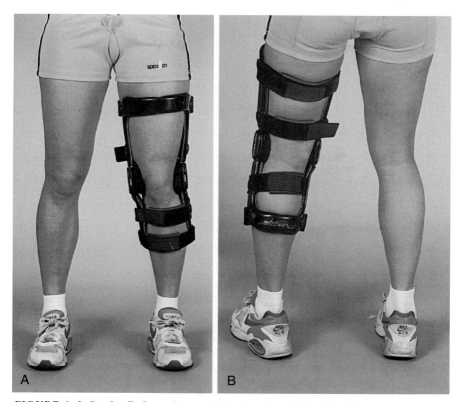

FIGURE 4–9. DonJoy Defiance Brace. *A*, Anterior view. *B*, Posterior view.

objective clinical testing in ACL-deficient knees. These patients exhibited a 100% improvement in the Lachman test and an 81% improvement in anterior drawer testing when the brace was worn. Reduction of clinical anterolateral rotatory instability was not as successful as assessed by elimination of the pivot shift sign. Only 33% of patients studied exhibited elimination of the pivot shift, 17% improved, and 50% showed no change. The authors concluded that the Lenox Hill Brace may be effective in decreasing anterolateral rotatory instability in knees with minor laxity problems.

Bodnar et al[3] reported on 100 patients with isolated ACL injuries. In this study, 40 patients wore a Lenox Hill Brace and 60 were unbraced. At an average 3-year follow-up evaluation, 40% of the braced group reported continued episodes of the knee's giving way compared to 60% of the unbraced patients. Perhaps an even more significant finding at follow-up was that 28% of the unbraced group suffered a meniscal tear sometime after the index cruciate ligament injury, compared to only 5% in the braced group. Retrospective analysis, however, did indicate a disproportionately higher percentage of patients with grade 3+ laxity among the unbraced patients.

Colville et al[8] demonstrated improved stability during instrumented liga-

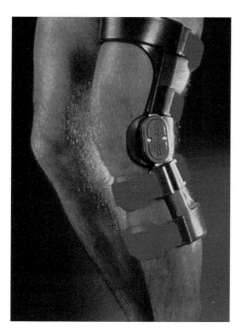

FIGURE 4-10. DonJoy CE2000 Brace. (Courtesy of Smith & Nephew DonJoy, Inc., Carlsbad, CA.)

ment testing in patients wearing a Lenox Hill Brace, although 62% of patients still reported functional instability. No decrease in anterior tibial translation associated with a maximal isolated quadriceps effort was measured, but a significant decrease in anterior shear force to an applied 100N force was noted. Seventy percent of patients felt the brace helped improve athletic performance. Forty percent of those individuals continued to wear the brace full-time, and 60% wore the brace for strenuous sports activities only. Twenty-two percent returned to preinjury sports without any brace, and 47% returned to preinjury sports using a brace. Approximately one quarter of the patients could not return to preinjury level of sports activity, but they felt that the brace was helpful. Nine percent were unable to return to a preinjury level of sports and felt that the brace was not helpful.[8]

Branch and Hunter[4] quoted a study presented in 1984 of 10 normal collegiate athletes. This study reported no functional differences in quadriceps and hamstring strength, 40-yard sprint speed, figure-eight running, or vertical jump height when the athletes were tested with and without a CTi Brace on one knee. A 1989 study found a 15% decrease in quadriceps EMG activity during stance phase of straight cutting and a 16% decrease in medial hamstring EMG activity when subjects were wearing either the CTi Brace or the Lenox Hill Brace.

A 1995 study by Stephens[21] revealed no significant effects on speed in collegiate athletes who were wearing the DonJoy GoldPoint Brace or the OMNI OS-5 Brace.

Generation II Unloader Brace for Medial Compartment Osteoarthritis

The Generation II Unloader Brace (Generation II Orthotics, Vancouver, British Columbia, Canada) is designed for patients with unicompartmental knee arthritis and can be fitted to decrease compressive forces on either the medial or the lateral joint surfaces. The high-carbon, Teflon-coated unilateral polyaxial hinge joins the steel shafts and is supported with a nylon strap (Fig. 4–11). This nylon strap places pressure either over the lateral aspect of the joint to unload the medial compartment, or over the medial aspect to decrease lateral joint pressure. The Generation II Unloader weighs approximately 26 ounces and is custom-made from a positive mold of the patient's knee.

Effectiveness in Clinical Trials

Pollo et al[17] measured a decreased external varus moment about the knee joint, during the midstance phase of gait, in nine subjects wearing the Generation II Unloader Brace for symptomatic medial compartment joint pain. Loomer and Horlick[15] reported a success rate of 82% in a group of 79

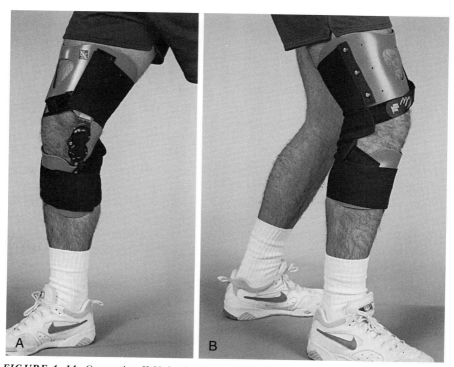

FIGURE 4–11. Generation II Unloader Brace. *A,* Medial view. *B,* Lateral view.

patients who were fitted with the Generation II Unloader Brace for medial joint osteoarthritis. At 20-month follow-up, 93% of those patients continued to wear the brace.

SUMMARY

Do prophylactic knee braces help decrease either the number or the severity of knee ligament (MCL or ACL) injuries in football players? Requa and Garrick[18] caution against drawing conclusions from laboratory studies performed on cadaver limbs under static conditions and generalizing those results to live athletes under dynamic conditions. Other concerns, such as the following, must be considered.

- Are injuries diagnosed correctly?
- Do different examiners classify the same injury similarly?
- Have any other rule changes been implemented that on their own may result in either fewer or more knee injuries?
- With what degree of certainty can the results of studies performed on college football players be relevant to decisions pertaining to high school or professional football players?

Manufacturers have made many claims concerning the biomechanical and technologic advances of knee braces. These claims of superior structure and function are based on sophisticated kinetics of hinge development, lighter and stronger materials affording the knee greater protection, and various straps and coutours designed to change the rotational torques about the injured joint.

Patients who require an orthosis to decrease ACL instability should be consulted regarding the choice of brace. A patient who does not like the style, texture, weight, or color of the orthosis will most likely not use it. Therefore, appropriate brace selection should result from input provided by the physician, physical therapist, athletic trainer, and patient.

Patients must also clearly understand the purpose of the functional brace. It is intended to provide additional protection and stability to the injured knee. At times, the cost of providing these benefits of knee protection will include sensations of decreased mobility or a cumbersome feeling. Commonly after a brace is fitted and paid for, patients remark that it feels awkward and interferes with sport activities.

Over the years, many of the following complaints regarding functional brace fit have been reported.

- Brace slippage—Patients with lean, muscular legs are more apt to have a brace that fits the knee properly and remains in place without any slippage. Others who lack optimal muscle tone and who have greater amounts of adipose tissue in the area to be braced may have a more difficult time obtaining a quality fit. When the patient is running or jumping, braces on these limbs may tend to migrate downward or even rotate slightly on the limb in knee positions near full extension. Fortunately, some braces come with neoprene undersleeves that may help minimize this problem.

- Bulkiness/weight—Many athletes feel that a bulky or heavy brace impairs functional performance. Braces of low weight are a strong selling point for brace companies.
- Heat retention/irritation—Heat retention and skin irritation are more prevalent problems in warmer climates or during the summer months. These problems are exacerbated by braces that utilize heavy straps. Heat rashes and underlying skin irritation can result.
- Excessive medial condylar tightness—Excessive medial condylar tightness is an occasional problem resulting in increased pressure and discomfort over the medial femoral condyle in relatively lean individuals. Patients may need to return the brace to the orthotist for alteration of the metal bars.
- Tightness of the calf strap—This phenomenon has been recognized primarily in larger male patients with a large calf circumference. The need to tighten the distal strap in order to adequately secure the brace has resulted in minor neurovascular complaints in the distal extremity.
- Brace hinge malalignment with condyles—Anterior or posterior migration of the brace hinges may increase either the flexion or the extension moment on the knee as it loses its normal alignment with the limb. Several instances have been reported in which the alignment of the brace does not match the position of the knee. The practitioner must be extremely aware of this problem in delicate ligament operations where extremes of range of motion must be avoided to allow healing. This author's experiences have suggested discrepancies of 10 to 15 degrees between the angle settings on the brace and the actual goniometric measurement of the joint.

REFERENCES

1. Anderson G, Seman SC, Rosenfeld RT: The Anderson knee stabler. Physician Sportsmed 7:125–127, 1979.
2. Bassett GS, Fleming BW: The Lenox Hill brace in anterolateral rotatory instability. Am J Sports Med 11:345–348, 1983.
3. Bodnar LM, Yergler DL, Bankorr DL, et al: Non-operative treatment of isolated anterior cruciate ligament injuries with the Lenox Hill brace. Presented at the AOSSM 10th Annual Meeting, Anaheim, CA, July 1984.
4. Branch TP, Hunter RE: Functional analysis of anterior cruciate ligament braces. Clin Sports Med 9:771–797, 1990.
5. Branch TP, Hunter R, Donath M: Dynamic EMG analysis of anterior cruciate deficient legs with and without bracing during cutting. Am J Sports Med 17:35–41, 1989.
6. Butler DL, Noyes FR, Grood ES: Ligamentous restraints to anterior-posterior drawer in the human knee. J Bone Joint Surg 62A:259–270, 1980.

7. Cawley PW, France EP, Paulos LE: Comparison of rehabilitative knee braces: A biomechanical investigation. Am J Sports Med 17:141–146, 1989.
8. Colville MR, Lee CL, Ciullo JV: The Lenox Hill brace: An evaluation of effectiveness in treating knee instability. Am J Sports Med 14:257–261, 1986.
9. Drez D, DeHaven K, D'Ambrosia R, et al: Knee Braces Seminar Report. American Academy of Orthopaedic Surgeons, Chicago, IL, 1984.
10. France EP, Paulos LE: In vitro assessment of prophylactic knee bracing. Clin Sports Med 9:823–841, 1990.
11. France EP, Paulos LE, Jayaraman G, et al: The biomechanics of lateral knee bracing II: Impact response of the braced knee. Am J Sports Med 15:430–438, 1987.
12. Grace TG, Skipper BJ, Newberry JC, et al: Prophylactic knee braces and injury to the lower extremity. J Bone Joint Surg 70A:422–427, 1988.
13. Hewson GF, Mendini RA, Wang JB: Prophylactic knee bracing in college football. Am J Sports Med 14:262–266, 1986.
14. Houston ME, Goemans PH: Leg muscle performance of athletes with and without knee support braces. Arch Phys Med Rehabil 63:431–432, 1982.
15. Loomer R, Horlick S: Valgus knee bracing for the osteoarthritic knee. Presented at the International Society of the Knee, Toronto, Ontario, Canada, May 1991.
16. Paulos LE, France EP, Rosenberg TD, et al: The biomechanics of lateral knee bracing, part I: Response of the valgus restraints to loading. Am J Sports Med 15:419–429, 1987.
17. Pollo FE, Otis JC, Wickiewicz TL, et al: Biomechanical analysis of valgus bracing for the osteoarthritic knee. Presented at the first North American Clinical Gait Lab Conference, Portland, OR, April 9, 1994.
18. Requa R, Garrick JG: Prophylactic knee brace studies in football. Clin Sports Med 9:853–869, 1990.
19. Rovere GD, Haupt HA, Yates CS: Prophylactic knee bracing in college football. Am J Sports Med 15:111–116, 1987.
20. Sitler MR, Ryan JR, Wheeler JG: The efficiency of a prophylactic knee brace to reduce knee injuries in football: A prospective randomized study. Proceedings of the American Orthopaedic Society for Sports Medicine, 15th Annual meeting, Traverse City, MI, June 21, 1989.
21. Stephens D: The effects of functional knee braces on speed in collegiate basketball players. J Orthop Sports Phys Ther 22:259–262, 1995.
22. Stevenson DV, Shields CL, Perry J, et al: Rehabilitative knee braces control of terminal extension in the ambulatory patient. Presented at the 34th Annual Meeting of the Orthopaedic Research Society, Atlanta, GA, February 1–4, 1988, p 517.
23. Teitz CC, Hermanson BK, Kronmal RA: Evaluation of the use of braces to prevent injury to the knee in college football players. J Bone Joint Surg 69A:2–9, 1987.
24. Wirth MA, DeLee JC: The history and classification of knee braces. Clin Sports Med, 9:731–741, 1990.
25. Zetterlund AE, Serfass RC, Hunter RE: The effect of wearing the complete Lenox Hill derotation brace on energy expenditure during horizontal treadmill running at 161 meters per minute. Am J Sports Med 14:73–76, 1986.

CHAPTER 5

Orthoses for the Ankle

MARCIA E. EPLER

The ankle joint has been the most frequently injured joint in athletics, comprising up to 25% of all time-loss injuries in running and jumping sports.[8, 27, 36, 38, 53, 72, 79, 84, 108, 122] One of every 17 individuals who participate in sports will sustain an injury to the ankle during the athletic season, and approximately 42% of those individuals with a prior history of ankle trauma will reinjure the joint.[8, 36, 108]

The primary purpose of an ankle support is to selectively limit movements of dorsiflexion, plantarflexion, inversion, and eversion to their respective physiologic extremes without compromising normal joint mechanics.[5, 13, 38, 45, 49, 56, 67, 122] Additional goals of orthoses and adhesive strappings at the ankle are to provide support and stability, as well as to enhance proprioceptive feedback and to facilitate muscular responses.[44]

This chapter presents the normal biomechanics and pathomechanics associated with ankle injury, the orthotic management strategies, and the effectiveness of clinical trials.

ANATOMY AND NORMAL MECHANICS

The major lateral ligamentous structures of the ankle include the anterior talofibular ligament (ATFL), the calcaneofibular ligament (CFL), and the posterior talofibular ligament (PTFL). The lateral ligaments provide lateral stability to the ankle dependent upon the position of the talus relative to the mortise (Fig. 5–1).[10, 20, 36, 58, 75, 115]

A cadaver study by Attarian et al[2] in 1985 determined the ATFL to be the weakest and most often injured of the lateral ligaments. The ATFL prevents

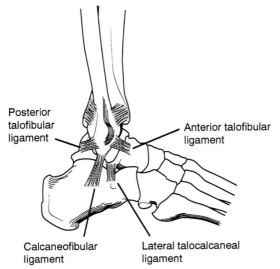

Posterior
talofibular
ligament

Anterior talofibular
ligament

Calcaneofibular
ligament

Lateral talocalcaneal
ligament

FIGURE 5–1. Lateral ligaments of the ankle.

excessive anterior displacement of the talus in the sagittal plane and counters varus stresses.[66] When the ankle is in a neutral position of dorsiflexion-plantarflexion, the fibers of the ATFL lie parallel to the long axis of the talus and, therefore, are not under stress. As ankle plantarflexion occurs, however, the ATFL becomes progressively tensed and assumes an orientation parallel to the axis of the leg allowing it to function somewhat as a collateral ligament.[3, 23] Therefore, the ATFL provides stability against excessive inversion forces when the foot is plantarflexed.[58, 75, 115]

The CFL, which has been reported to be 2.5 times stronger than the ATFL, crosses both the talocrural and talocalcaneal joints. The function of the CFL is to prevent inversion of the talus and calcaneus during a varus stress.[2, 66] The CFL is oriented almost perpendicular to the long axis of the talus when the ankle is in a neutral position of dorsiflexion-plantarflexion. The CFL provides stability against inversion forces with the foot in a dorsiflexed position.[58, 75, 115] Progressive plantarflexion causes a relaxation of the CFL fibers.[23] It is evident from these mechanical descriptions that the ATFL and CFL function synergistically: while one ligament is relaxed, the other remains taut.[106]

The strongest and least frequently injured of the lateral ligaments is the posterior talofibular ligament. Its fibers are oriented nearly horizontally and are stressed only in extreme dorsiflexion.[66] The function of the PTFL is to assist in the resistance of anterior leg dislocation relative to the foot.[58, 75, 115]

The medially located deltoid ligament is the strongest of all the collateral ligaments and functions to provide medial stability to the ankle (Fig. 5–2). The deltoid ligament can be subdivided into four portions: the tibionavicular portion, which lies anterior and superficial; the anterior tibiotalar portion,

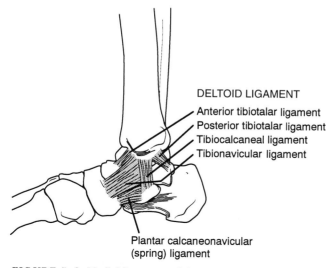

DELTOID LIGAMENT
Anterior tibiotalar ligament
Posterior tibiotalar ligament
Tibiocalcaneal ligament
Tibionavicular ligament

Plantar calcaneonavicular
(spring) ligament

FIGURE 5–2. Medial ligaments of the ankle.

which lies anterior and deep; the tibiocalcaneal portion, which runs posterior and superficial; and the posterior tibiotalar portion, which runs posterior and deep.[65] Ankle dorsiflexion is, in part, restricted by the posterior fibers of the CFL laterally and the deltoid ligament medially. Conversely, ankle plantarflexion is partly limited by the anterior fibers of the deltoid medially and the ATFL laterally.[57]

Under dynamic loading, the deltoid ligament sustains the highest load prior to failure, whereas the ATFL possesses the lowest tensile strength of all the major ankle ligaments. The tensile strengths of the CFL and PTFL lie between those of the ATF and deltoid ligaments.[65]

PATHOMECHANICS AND MECHANISMS OF INJURY

Ankle sprains are the most commonly sustained injuries in physically active individuals, with the plantarflexion inversion mechanism being most prevalent.[3, 7, 30, 35, 37, 38, 59, 79, 89, 95] Various studies have demonstrated that isolated injuries to the ATFL constitute two thirds of all ankle sprains.[10, 12, 74] Sprains to the medial and lateral ligamentous structures occur in a weight-bearing position when movements of the ankle exceed normal physiologic movement capacities.[20, 38, 42, 64, 65, 115] A study reported that the articular surfaces, rather than actual ligamentous integrity, provide stability to the ankle during weight-bearing activities.[116] Stormont et al[116] determined that during physiologic weight bearing, the articular bony restraints accounted for 30% and 100% of joint stability during rotation and inversion-eversion movements, respectively. This finding raises the question whether some instances of ankle instability may result from rotational movements rather than from excessive inversion stresses. The common plantarflexion inversion sprain occurs during plantar flexion and inversion of the weight-bearing foot as the tibia externally rotates.[12, 114] During a plantarflexion inversion injury, the anterolateral capsule is the initial structure torn, followed by the ATFL and the anterior tibiofibular ligaments. Following complete rupture of the ATFL, progressive inversion causes the fibers of the CFL to be injured, and ultimately the PTFL may be involved. The isolated CFL injury may occur with the ankle in a more neutral position because of the perpendicular orientation of the ligamentous fibers. Injuries to both the ATFL and the CFL frequently result in lateral instability, regardless of the ankle position.[65] The PTFL, which prevents posterior displacement of the talus relative to the leg, is rarely injured. Excessive amounts of force may also result in damage to the deltoid ligament medially.[12, 23, 42, 114, 115]

The less common incidence of eversion sprains can be explained partly by the anatomic constraints of the joint. Calcaneal eversion motion is less than that of inversion because of the distal projection of the lateral malleolus of the fibula. Additionally, the broad, expansive deltoid ligament is better suited to resist tensile forces than the lateral ligamentous structures.[25, 64] The eversion sprain occurs with dorsiflexion and eversion of the weight-bearing foot in conjunction with tibial internal rotation. These forces result in tearing of the deltoid ligament, the anterior tibiofibular ligament, and the interosseous membrane.[52] In addition, excessive eversion forces, limited by the anatomic bony block, may be associated with compression fractures of the fibula, with high ankle sprains, with avulsion of a bony fragment of the medial malleolus, and with fracture dislocation of the ankle joint.[57, 65]

The peroneal muscles and ankle mechanoreceptors play an important role in lateral joint stability. In one study, more than 50% of patients with a history of repeated ankle sprains exhibited weakness of the peroneal muscles rather than ligamentous laxity.[76] Additionally, denervation potentials of the peroneal nerve may be present up to 6 months following injury.[98] Freeman et al[31] in 1965, suggested that injury to the lateral ligaments is accompanied by damage to the mechanoreceptors, resulting in deficiencies in ankle proprioception. A resultant loss of normal sensory input from the mechano-receptors may be responsible for increasing the risk of reinjury due to abnormal ankle posturing and decreased postural reflex responses.[31] More recent evidence has suggested that muscle receptors, not joint receptors, may provide the primary input for joint position sense.[14, 46] Repetitive ankle sprains may occur because of an alteration of position sense and postural reflexes associated with the initial injury.[31] A patient with a history of re-peated ankle sprains exhibits not only ligamentous laxity but also damage to sensory receptors located in the joint capsule and surrounding muscle tissue.[46, 96]

Some researchers have reported an increase in postural sway associated with recurrent ankle sprains, owing to the injury and disruption of the joint proprioceptors.[34, 39, 123, 124] Several studies have investigated the relationship of unilateral postural sway between injured and noninjured ankles. In a 1965 study of individuals with an injured ankle, Freeman et al[31] reported that patients experienced an increased amount of unilateral postural sway while balancing on the injured lower limb. Garn and Newton,[34] in 1988, also documented deficits of balance on the side of the injured ankle as compared to the normal ankle. Conversely, in 1985, Tropp et al[124] found no significant difference in the amplitude of unilateral postural sway between injured and noninjured ankles of patients studied.

RATIONALE FOR USE

The overall objectives of orthotic management include the prevention or correction of deformity, the support or immobilization of a body segment, and the assistance or restoration of mobility and function.[105]

The prophylactic or postinjury selection of orthoses over adhesive tape has been advantageous. Orthotic intervention is more cost-effective than the repeated application of adhesive tape. Additionally, the application of tape often requires the assistance of another person, and is associated with skin irritation and breakdown, and tape loosens significantly shortly after use.[32, 49, 56, 87, 104, 107]

TYPES OF ORTHOSES

Ankle stabilizers have been categorized as softshell or semirigid. The first softshell ankle orthoses, constructed of materials such as canvas (Fig. 5–3) and neoprene rubber, were introduced in the early 1980s.[83] The first non-commercial semirigid ankle supports were fabricated in 1974 with Orthoplast (J & J Skillman, NJ); the commercial semirigid stabilizers were introduced by Aircast (Aircast, Inc., Summit, NJ) in 1980.[59, 117] Table 5–1 lists the softshell ankle orthoses, and Table 5–2 lists the semirigid orthoses. Although there are many ankle supports available on the market, the braces described in these two tables have been limited to those discussed in the literature.

EFFECTIVENESS IN CLINICAL TRIALS

Several clinical studies have been conducted to date in an attempt to establish the efficacy of ankle orthoses. The studies reviewed in this section are organized according to the various selection criteria for which a specific ankle orthosis may be chosen. These selection criteria include prophylaxis, effects on range of motion and torque production, effect on functional

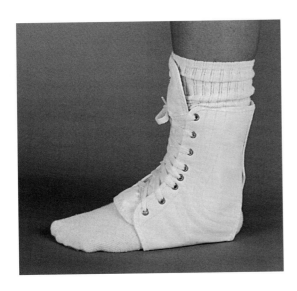

FIGURE 5–3. Mueller ATF Brace. (Courtesy of Mueller Sports Medicine, Prairie du Sac, WI.)

TABLE 5-1
Softshell Ankle Orthoses

Orthoses	Design Characteristics	Function	Studies
ASO Ankle Stabilizing Orthoses	Thin, durable ballistic nylon slip-on secured by laces Nonstretch nylon heel lock straps	Restricts inversion-eversion	
Donjoy RocketSoc	Neoprene rubber Slides over ankle with opening anterior to talocrural joint Three Velcro straps for support	Restricts inversion-eversion	Range of motion and torque production
Kallassy	Nylon-lined neoprene sleeve Two lateral nonelastic Velcro straps One medial nonelastic strap	Restricts inversion and limits midfoot/rearfoot motion	Range of motion and torque production, functional performance, patient assessment
McDavid Ankle Guard	Canvas-like material Slip-on with anterior laces	Restricts inversion-eversion	Range of motion and torque production, functional performance
Mueller ATF	Canvas material with lining Slip-on lacing system ATF strap over course of ligament Flexible steel springs medial and lateral	Restricts inversion-eversion	
Omni Duo-Loc	Canvas material Slip-on with anterior laces Nonelastic "duo-loc" strap for heel lock	Provides rearfoot/forefoot stability Restricts inversion-eversion	
Swede-O-Universal	Double layer of canvas Slip-on with anterior laces Medial and lateral panels Optional medial and lateral plastic inserts	Restricts inversion-eversion Limits midfoot/rearfoot motion	Range of motion and torque production, functional performance, patient assessment

TABLE 5–2
Semirigid Ankle Orthoses

Orthoses	Design Characteristics	Function	Studies
Active Ankle	Bilateral thermoplastic shells in U-shape. Shells lined with molded adjustable pads. Bilateral hinge joints aligned with ankle. Two straps over lower leg; one strap over Achilles	Restricts inversion-eversion	Range of motion and torque production, functional performance
Aircast Air-Stirrup	Medial and lateral thermoplastic shells with inflatable air cells. Two Velcro straps to secure brace to lower leg	Restricts inversion-eversion	Range of motion and torque production, functional performance, early mobilization, patient assessment
Aircast Standard Ankle	Same as Air-Stirrup	Restricts inversion-eversion. Recommended following acute injury	Balance and proprioception
Aircast Ankle Training	Same as Air-Stirrup but 25% smaller	Restricts inversion-eversion. Recommended for chronic instability, prophylaxis, and acute injury in smaller patient	Range of motion and torque production, functional performance, patient assessment
Aircast Sport-Stirrup	Same as Air-Stirrup but smaller and more contoured shells over malleoli	Restricts inversion-eversion. Recommended for prophylaxis	Prophylaxis, range of motion and torque production, functional performance
Donjoy ALP	Injection-molded plastic polymers. Calf cuff with Velcro closure. Posterior vertical support between calf cuff and heel cup. Distal plastic heel cup attached to shoe	Restricts inversion-eversion. Transfers force from heel to tibia	Range of motion and torque production, functional performance, patient assessment
Gelcast	Medial and lateral plastic shells with gel-filled sacs. Velcro straps to secure brace to leg	Restricts inversion-eversion	Range of motion and torque production
Malleoloc	Single U-shaped plastic mold lined with padding anterior and posterior to lateral and medial malleolus. Three color-coded Velcro straps	Restricts inversion-eversion	Range of motion and torque production, patient assessment

performance, balance and proprioceptive input, early mobilization effects, and patient assessment. All reported differences were statistically significant unless otherwise stated.

Prophylaxis

Two published studies have assessed the prophylactic effectiveness of ankle orthoses. Sitler and associates[112] investigated the effect of wearing an Aircast Sport-Stirrup (Aircast, Inc., Summit, NJ) in conjunction with high-top shoes in 1601 cadets at the United States Military Academy (Fig. 5–4). Cadets wearing the Sport-Stirrup in conjunction with the high-top shoes suffered fewer injuries to the ATFL and CFL than did cadets wearing the high-top shoes only. Additionally, no increase in the incidence of knee injuries was associated with wearing the ankle orthosis. The incidence of noncontact ankle injuries did not significantly differ between the groups. Conversely, a significant difference was observed in those with contact injuries, in that cadets using the ankle orthosis sustained fewer injuries than cadets wearing shoes only.

In 1994 Surve et al[120] investigated the efficacy of the Aircast Sport-Stirrup in the prevention of recurrent ankle sprains in 258 soccer players with previous ankle sprains and in 246 players with no history of ankle injury. The Sport-Stirrup reduced the number and severity of sprains in those players with a history of prior injury, but it had no significant effect on the incidence of injury in players with no history of ankle sprains.

Range-of-Motion Limitation Studies

Various commercially available braces have been studied with respect to their ability to restrict the ankle from moving beyond the limits of its normal,

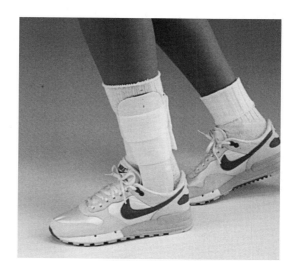

FIGURE 5–4. Aircast Sport-Stirrup Brace. (Courtesy of Aircast, Inc., Summit, NJ.)

physiologic range of motion (ROM). Because of the large number of clinical studies that have investigated the effect of ankle orthoses on ROM, the following section is organized according to the braces studied.

SWEDE-O-UNIVERSAL. The softshell Swede-O-Universal (Swede-O-Universal, Inc., North Branch, MN) ankle support was reported to be ineffective in limiting talar tilt in subjects with a history of ankle injury[16] (Fig. 5–5). A 1995 study by Paris and associates[101] demonstrated that ankle plantarflexion ROM increased after 15 minutes of activity with the Sub-Talar Support Brace (Sport-Mate Services, LTD, Mississauga, Ontario, Canada) and after 30 minutes with the Swede-O-Universal support. Both ankle supports demonstrated increased ankle inversion after 15 minutes of exercise. Overall, the Swede-O-Universal Ankle Brace provided greater support compared with the Sub-Talar Support Brace.

AIRCAST AIR-STIRRUP. The ability of the Aircast Air-Stirrup to control a sudden induced weight-bearing ankle inversion stress was investigated by Kimura et al[67] in 1987. The use of the Air-Stirrup was associated with less ankle inversion ROM than that found in unbraced, control ankles[67] (Fig. 5–6). In comparisons with adhesive tape, the Aircast ankle orthoses have consistently been more effective in controlling ankle inversion-eversion ROM. Hughes and Stetts[56] reported no difference in inversion ROM following application of either ankle tape or the Aircast Sport-Stirrup. After 20 minutes of exercise, however, both the ankles with the Aircast Sport-Stirrup and those with adhesive strapping demonstrated a comparable decreased ability to restrict inversion as compared with pre-exercise values.[56] Gross and associates[49] reported significant restriction of the total inversion-

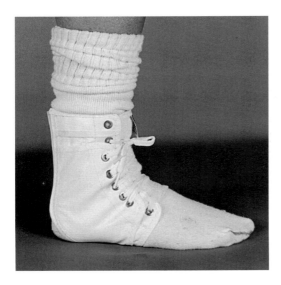

FIGURE 5–5. Swede-O-Universal Brace. (Courtesy of Swede-O-Universal, Inc., North Branch, MN.)

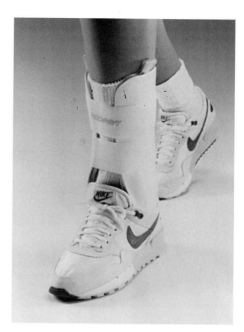

FIGURE 5–6. Aircast Standard Ankle Brace. (Courtesy of Aircast, Inc., Summit, NJ.)

eversion ROM following application of adhesive tape and the Aircast Air-Stirrup, with the Aircast being more restrictive than the tape. This finding was attributed to a greater restriction of eversion compared with that provided by the tape. Following exercise, both supports continued to restrict both inversion and eversion ROM, although loosening in inversion was observed in the taped ankles.[49] A 1994 study by Mack and associates[80] demonstrated restriction of ankle inversion following tape application, but this restrictive capability was lost following exercise. Conversely, the Aircast Sport-Stirrup reduced the amount of inversion after application and continued to maintain its support after exercise.[80]

DONJOY ALP. The effect of the DonJoy ALP (Smith & Nephew DonJoy, Inc., Carlsbad, CA) ankle orthoses in restricting ankle mobility has been investigated by various researchers (Fig. 5–7). Greene and Roland[44] reported in 1989 that the ALP orthosis limited active inversion and eversion ROM, with a mean decrease of 30.16% in total inversion-eversion ROM compared with the unbraced trials. Following 20 minutes of exercise, a slight nonsignificant decrease in the ability to limit ROM was observed when these findings were compared with pre-exercise values. No differences in peak torque were generated between nonbraced and ALP conditions, indicating that the orthosis did not inhibit the production of torque. Interestingly, 26% and 23% of the braced subjects demonstrated greater torque output in eversion and inversion, respectively, when compared with nonbraced

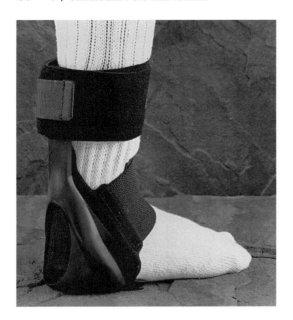

FIGURE 5-7. DonJoy ALP Brace. (Courtesy of Smith & Nephew DonJoy, Inc., Carlsbad, CA.)

subjects.[44] A study by Greene and Hillman[43] in 1990 compared inversion-eversion support provided by the DonJoy ALP before, during, and after 3 hours of volleyball practice. Application of the DonJoy ALP limited inversion-eversion ROM by approximately 40%. Following 60 minutes of exercise, there was no loosening in inversion and eversion while the athletes were wearing the brace. Following 90 minutes of exercise, no loss of inversion restriction was evident in the braced ankles, but eversion ROM increased. Additionally, vertical jump ability was not affected by either treatment.[43] Gross and associates[48] in 1994 reported eversion ROM to be reduced, compared with preapplication levels, following application of the DonJoy ALP and a subtalar sling. Eversion ROM increased following exercise with both supports, but both continued to provide eversion limitations over preapplication values. The subtalar sling provided greater limitation to ankle inversion than the ALP after application, but the ability to restrict inversion with the subtalar sling was compromised following exercise. Compared with preapplication ROM, inversion was restricted by the ALP following both application and exercise. Overall, the amount of inversion restriction after exercise was similar in both supports.[48]

AIRCAST AIR-STIRRUP AND SWEDE-O-UNIVERSAL. Some authors investigated the differences between the semirigid Aircast ankle orthoses and the softshell Swede-O-Universal support. A 1991 study by Gross and colleagues[51] reported a difference in the amount of eversion ROM available after application of the Aircast Air-Stirrup, the Swede-O-Universal, and adhesive tape. The Air-

Stirrup provided the greatest limitation to ankle eversion. The Swede-O-Universal and athletic tape followed with an equal ability to restrict eversion. Following exercise, the amount of eversion motion was similar for the support devices, but all the orthoses exhibited some degree of loosening. The amount of eversion allowable in all three supports remained restrictive, however, relative to preapplication values. Each of the supports equally restricted ankle inversion following application, with tape being more restrictive than either the Air-Stirrup or the Swede-O-Universal. All support devices continued to provide inversion support after exercise, but the degree of support was not symmetric between devices. The Air-Stirrup and adhesive strapping were equitable in the amount of inversion restriction after exercise and were better able to limit inversion than the Swede-O-Universal. The tape loosened significantly after exercise, however, allowing more inversion than occurred before exercise.[51] In 1993, Martin and Harter[87] found that active ankle inversion ROM was equally restricted when a person was wearing either the Aircast Sport-Stirrup or the Swede-O-Universal ankle supports. Adhesive strapping of the ankle was not as effective as wearing either of the other orthoses. Following an exercise program, the subjects wearing the Sport-Stirrup Ankle Support experienced restricted inversion, but the unbraced control group did not. Both the Swede-O-Universal and Sport-Stirrup were similarly effective in allowing significantly less inversion ROM than that found in the control group during running. The adhesive tape provided the least amount of support before and after all exercise sessions and loosened the most.[87]

Paris and Jones[100] in 1994 demonstrated that the Aircast Air-Stirrup, the Swede-O-Universal, and the subtalar supports all reduced inversion-eversion ROM compared to presupport levels with the ankle in both a neutral and a plantarflexed position. With the ankle in a neutral position, inversion range increased with the Air-Stirrup following 20 minutes of exercise, but this increase was not observed until after 60 minutes of exercise with the Swede-O-Universal and the subtalar supports. Increases in eversion motion were reported with the Air-Stirrup and the Swede-O-Universal braces at the 40-minute testing interval and with the subtalar support following 60 minutes of exercise. With the ankle in 20 degrees of plantarflexion, the Air-Stirrup and subtalar support demonstrated increased inversion at the 60-minute exercise interval and increased eversion at the 40- and 60-minute sessions, respectively. The range of ankle inversion-eversion was unaffected by exercise while subjects were wearing the Swede-O-Universal support.[100]

AIRCAST AIR-STIRRUP AND DONJOY ALP. Comparisons between two semirigid ankle orthoses, namely the Aircast and the DonJoy ALP, have been studied by one clinical investigator. A 1992 study by Gross and associates[47] demonstrated ankle eversion ROM to be reduced when subjects were wearing the Aircast Air-Stirrup and DonJoy ALP braces. Additionally, both braces restricted inversion after both application and exercise, with the

DonJoy ALP being more restrictive than the Air-Stirrup. Both orthoses were equally effective in limiting eversion following application but allowed more eversion following exercise.[47]

ELASTIC SUPPORTS. In a 1984 study of elastic supports, Myburgh et al[94] reported that neither the Ace guard nor the Futuroguard provided support for any ankle movements before, during, or after exercise.

MIKROS 7″ CRAMER STABILIZER AND ANK-L-AID. In 1985 Bunch et al[13] compared the ankle support offered by reusable lace-on braces with that offered by conventional ankle strapping. Analysis indicated that adhesive tape provided the greatest amount of support, being 25% stiffer than the optimal laced device and 70% stiffer than a cotton wrap. The Mikros 7″ Cramer Stabilizer (Cramer Products, Inc., Gardner, KS) and Ank-L-Aid (Ank-L-Aid, Inc., Ardmore, PA) did not differ from the cotton wrap in support. The Mikros 9″ and Swede-O-Universal were more supportive than the cotton wrap, but less supportive than the adhesive tape. Following exercise, however, subjects wearing adhesive tape demonstrated a 21% loss of support. Only a 4.5% to 8.5% loss of support occurred with the lace-on braces. No difference was observed in the support provided by the tape, the Swede-O-Universal Brace, and the Mikros 9″ Stabilizer.

AIRCAST AIR-STIRRUP, DONJOY ALP, AND SWEDE-O-UNIVERSAL. Greene and Wright[45] reported in 1990 that the Aircast Air-Stirrup, the DonJoy ALP, and the Swede-O-Universal orthoses all restricted the total inversion-eversion ROM. Total ROM was limited by 42.92% with the ALP, by 42.02% with the Air-Stirrup, and by 30.84% with the Swede-O-Universal. After 20 minutes of exercise, the support provided by the Swede-O-Universal was compromised in both inversion and eversion ranges. The inversion-eversion support was further diminished after subjects played 40 minutes of softball, and even less range restriction into inversion was evident after 60 minutes of play. No loosening of the Air-Stirrup or ALP was found following both 20 and 40 minutes of softball. After 90 minutes of play, the Air-Stirrup loosened in inversion, but no loss of eversion restriction occurred. No loss of support was noted in the group wearing the DonJoy ALP. Functionally, the DonJoy ALP and the Swede-O-Universal had no effect on base running ability, whereas the Air-Stirrup slightly diminished base running ability.

AIRCAST AIR-STIRRUP, SWEDE-O-UNIVERSAL, AND ACTIVE ANKLE. Gehlsen and associates[40] determined in 1991 that the amount of dorsiflexion ROM in the unbraced control group was greater than the amount in the group wearing the Aircast Air-Stirrup, the tape, and the Swede-O-Universal supports; however, this difference was not significant for persons using the Active Ankle orthosis (Active Ankle Systems, Inc., Louisville, KY) (Fig. 5–8). The Active Ankle and Aircast Air-Stirrup were optimal for approximating full

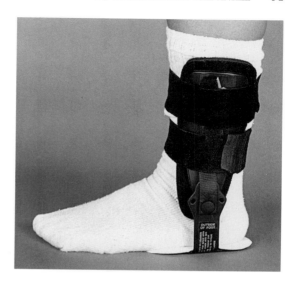

FIGURE 5–8. Active Ankle Brace. (Courtesy of Active Ankle Systems, Inc., Louisville, KY.)

ankle dorsiflexion-plantarflexion ROM. The Swede-O-Universal and adhesive strapping restricted dorsiflexion-plantarflexion ROM. Plantarflexion peak torque at 30 and 120 degrees per second decreased 11% to 19% compared to the nonsupport condition in the group wearing the Air-Stirrup, the Active Ankle, the tape, and the Swede-O-Universal supports. At 180 degrees per second, plantarflexion peak torque was diminished 9% to 21% over the control in those persons wearing the Air-Stirrup, the tape, and the Swede-O-Universal supports. Conversely, the Active Ankle group exhibited a 7.8% increase in plantarflexion peak torque over the control group. Dorsiflexion peak torque was not different when all treatments and the control were compared. No difference in dorsiflexion work between the control and the support conditions was observed; however, the control trial produced 4% to 24% more plantarflexion work than the support conditions.

AIRCAST AIR-STIRRUP, KALLASSY, DONJOY ALP, AND SWEDE-O-UNIVERSAL. Alves et al[1] demonstrated in 1992 that application of the Kallassy Ankle Support (Sports Supports, Dallas, TX), the DonJoy ALP, the Swede-O-Universal Ankle Support, and the Aircast Air-Stirrup limited the total allowable inversion-eversion ROM by at least 18% (Fig. 5–9). The Air-Stirrup provided the most restriction of total movement at 29%, followed by the DonJoy ALP at 27%, the Swede-O-Universal at 21%, and the Kallassy at 18%. After subjects had exercised for 10 minutes, all orthoses were able to restrict total movement by at least 12%, with the Air-Stirrup again most limiting at 27%. This restrictive capability was measured for the DonJoy ALP at 25%, the Swede-O-Universal at 15%, and the Kallassy at 12%. The difference in total inversion-eversion motion between pre- and postexercise levels was insignificant for the Air-Stirrup and the DonJoy ALP, but loosening was

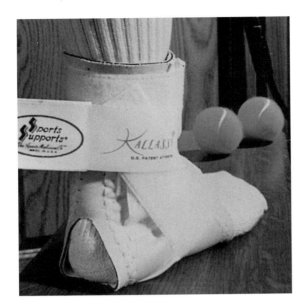

FIGURE 5-9. Kallassy Brace. (Courtesy of Sports Supports, Dallas, TX.)

noted with the Kallassy and Swede-O-Universal supports. No difference was found between the semirigid Air-Stirrup and the DonJoy ALP orthoses in the ability to control total ROM, but the softshell Swede-O-Universal restricted inversion-eversion better than the Kallassy.[1]

ACTIVE ANKLE, AIRCAST AIR-STIRRUP, AND DONJOY ALP. Lindley and Kernozek[77] reported in 1995 that the maximal plantarflexion allowed by the DonJoy ALP was less than that offered by the Active Ankle "Trainer" orthosis, Air-Stirrup "Training" orthosis, and adhesive tape (Fig. 5–10).

Maximal plantarflexion ROM was observed at toe-off under all conditions of support. The point in the gait cycle where maximal dorsiflexion occurred varied among subjects from initial contact to just prior to heel-off. No difference in maximal dorsiflexion was observed among the devices tested. The functional dorsiflexion-plantarflexion ROM allowed by the DonJoy ALP (25 degrees) was less than that measured for the other three conditions. The functional ROM for the ankles with the DonJoy ALP was 17% less than that for the unbraced control and 13% less than the ROM with the Air-Stirrup, the Active Ankle, and the tape. The functional ROM, observed during closed chain assessment, was 29.3 degrees in the Active Ankle device and 28.6 degrees in the Air-Stirrup device. The overall mean functional ROM in this study was 30.2 degrees at an average velocity of 6.4 meters per second.

AIRCAST AIR-STIRRUP, ACTIVE ANKLE, MALLEOLOC, AND DONJOY ALP. Johnson and colleagues[62] observed in 1994 that the Aircast Air-Stirrup and the Active Ankle braces were similar in restricting inversion ROM following brace

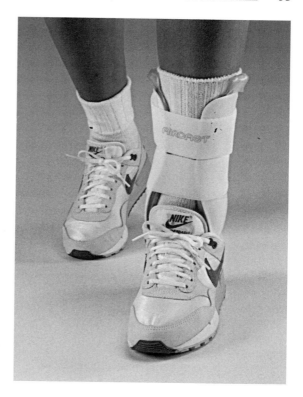

FIGURE 5–10. Aircast Ankle Training Brace. (Courtesy of Aircast, Inc., Summit, NJ.)

application and exercise compared to the Malleoloc (Bauerfeind, USA, Inc., Kennesaw, GA) and the DonJoy ALP (Fig. 5–11). The DonJoy ALP limited ankle inversion more than the Malleoloc both before and after exercise. All four ankle supports revealed a 3.27-degree increase in inversion ROM between preexercise and postexercise levels.

McDAVID ANKLE GUARD A-101, AIRCAST AIR-STIRRUP, GELCAST, PRO SUPER-8, DONJOY FG-062, ECLIPSE EXCEL, CRAMER ANKLE STABILIZER, AND HIGH-TOP ANKLE SUPPORT. In a 1994 study of five cadaver ankles, Shapiro et al[111] reported that the McDavid Ankle Guard A-101 (McDavid, Inc., Clarendon Hills, IL), the Air-Stirrup Training Brace, the Gelcast (Centec Orthopedics, Division of Royce Medical Co., Agorra Hills, CA), the Super-8 (Pro Orthopedic Devices, Inc., Tucson, AZ), the DonJoy Model FG-062 (Smith & Nephew DonJoy, Inc., Carlsbad, CA), the Eclipse Excel Ankle Support (Surefit Orthopedics, Culver City, CA), the Ankle Stabilizer (Cramer Products, Inc., Gardner, KS), and the High-Top Ankle Support (Technol Products, Inc., Fort Worth, TX) provided resistance to an inversion moment. All ankle supports provided greater than twice the amount of resistance to the inversion force, with the Super-8 brace being superior. In all test scenarios, with the exception of the

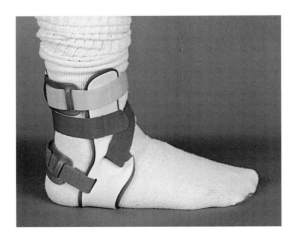

FIGURE 5–11. Malleoloc Brace. (Courtesy of Bauerfeind, USA, Inc., Kennesaw, GA.)

unprotected ankle, a greater amount of force was required to invert the ankle while the foot was in a neutrally dorsiflexed position than that required for 30 degrees of plantarflexion. When the foot was wearing a low-top shoe, all orthoses stiffened the unprotected ankle. Wearing a high-top shoe maximized protection of an ankle, in that the high-top shoe doubled the inversion resistance whether the ankle was plantarflexed or neutral. No difference was observed between the braces or the tape in the resistance to inversion when a high-top shoe was worn. The Air-Stirrup, the DonJoy, and the Gelcast increased the resistance to inversion when high-top shoes were worn in both positions of testing. The inversion resistance provided by the Cramer orthosis, although not significant, was less than or equal to that provided by the taped ankle under all conditions tested.

Functional Performance Studies

The effect of various ankle orthoses on functional performance has been the focus of many clinical studies. As in the previous section, this portion of the chapter is organized according to specific braces studied.

McDAVID A-101, NEW CROSS #120, AND SWEDE-O-UNIVERSAL. Some investigators have reported that ankle orthoses have little, if any, negative effect on functional performance. Paris[99] demonstrated in 1992 that activities involving speed, balance, and agility were not affected under conditions of wearing tape support, the McDavid A-101 ankle brace, the New Cross #120 ankle support (New Cross International Limited, Scarborough, Ontario, Canada), and the Swede-O-Universal ankle support. Vertical jump height was compromised when athletes wore the New Cross ankle brace only.

ACTIVE ANKLE TRAINING AND AIRCAST AIR-STIRRUP. A 1994 study by Bocchinfuso et al[9] reported that neither the Active Ankle Training Brace nor the Aircast Air-Stirrup had an effect on a vertical jump, a shuttle run, an 80-foot sprint, or a four-point run. Some trends, although not significant, were noted in that the Air-Stirrup improved performance in the shuttle run and four-point run compared to the unsupported or Active Ankle conditions.

AIRCAST AIR-STIRRUP AND DONJOY ALP. Gross and colleagues[50] observed in 1994 that neither the DonJoy ALP nor the Aircast Air-Stirrup orthoses had an effect on a 40-meter sprint, a figure-eight run, or a standing vertical jump.

AIRCAST TRAINING, AIRCAST SPORT-STIRRUP, DONJOY ALP, AND SWEDE-O-UNIVERSAL. In a 1994 study, Beriau and associates[6] found no differences in the ability of an athlete to run an agility course under braced conditions of the Swede-O-Universal, the Aircast Training Brace, the Aircast Sport-Stirrup, or the DonJoy ALP when compared to the ability under unbraced trials. Athletes wearing the DonJoy ALP, however, exhibited a slower time for completion of the agility course than those wearing the Aircast Training Brace.

AIRCAST SPORT-STIRRUP AND DONJOY ROCKETSOC. MacPherson and associates[83] reported in 1995 that neither the Aircast Sport-Stirrup nor the RocketSoc (Smith & Nephew DonJoy, Inc., Carlsbad, CA) had an effect on an athlete's ability to perform a 40-yard spring, a 20-yard shuttle run, or a vertical jump (Fig. 5–12). However, skill players demonstrated faster 40-yard sprint times compared to strength players under all conditions of ankle support.[83]

SWEDE-O-UNIVERSAL AND KALLASSY. A 1991 study by Burks and associates[15] reported that functional performance was negatively affected under all conditions of ankle support including the Swede-O-Universal, the Kallassy brace, and adhesive strapping. The taping condition slightly reduced the height of the vertical jump by 4%, the shuttle run time by 1.6%, and the sprint time by 3.5%. The distance of the broad jump was also lessened, but this difference was not significant. The time to complete the shuttle run was not altered when subjects wore the Swede-O-Universal support, but sprint time was reduced by 3.2%, broad jump distance was shortened by 3.6%, and vertical jump height was lessened by 4.6%. The Kallassy Brace only affected the vertical jump height by 3.4%. Differences in the shuttle run, sprint, and broad jump were not significant. With respect to performance, the two ankle supports were not different, with the exception of the broad jump distance's being shortened with the Swede-O-Universal compared with the Kallassy Brace. Additionally, the time to completion in the shuttle run was slower with the taped ankles compared to the time with the Kallassy Brace.

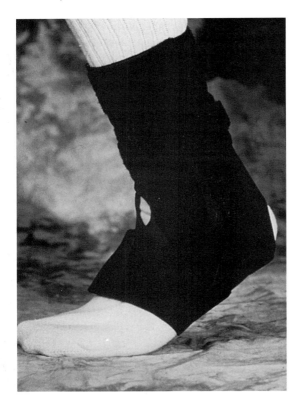

FIGURE 5–12. DonJoy Roc-ketSoc. (Courtesy of Smith & Nephew DonJoy, Inc., Carlsbad, CA.)

ACTIVE ANKLE, AIRCAST AIR-STIRRUP, AND SWEDE-O-UNIVERSAL. MacKean et al[81] observed in 1995 that the highest performance level overall was attained with no ankle support at all, followed in order by the Active Ankle, tape, the Aircast Air-Stirrup, and the Swede-O-Universal supports. A detrimental effect was observed under all conditions of ankle support when compared to the unbraced control trials, but no differences were evident between the brace types. Additionally, no differences in sprint time were seen regardless of the ankle support worn.

AIRCAST AIR-STIRRUP TRAINING, KALLASSY, AND SWEDE-O-UNIVERSAL. A 1995 study by Pienkowski et al[102] determined that neither the Aircast Air-Stirrup Training, the Kallassy, nor the Swede-O-Universal ankle support had an effect on vertical jump, standing long jump, cone running, or an 18.3-meter shuttle run.

Proprioception and Balance Studies

An early study by Stuessi et al[119] in 1985 reported that wearing the Aircast decreased the amount of both static and running (dynamic) supination at the foot compared with wearing solely a running shoe. In addition, the Aircast ankle brace had no effect on the EMG activity of the peroneal muscles, suggesting that limitation of supination resulted from the brace and not from enhanced muscular contraction.

In 1993 Feuerbach and Grabiner[28] observed no differences between the right and left lower limb stance, except that static anterior-posterior sway amplitude was decreased compared to unbraced trial results. The anterior-posterior static postural sway did not differ in frequency or in the tendency to shift body weight between braced and unbraced trials. The medial-lateral static postural sway amplitude and frequency were decreased while the Aircast was worn compared to the nonbraced ankle condition. Subjects also exhibited a trend toward lateral weight shifting of the body while wearing the Aircast. During testing of postural sway under dynamic conditions, the medial-lateral sway amplitude was not very different between the Aircast and control conditions, but the frequency of sway was decreased with the Aircast. There was also a trend, as seen statically, to shift the body weight laterally. Dynamic assessment of anterior-posterior postural sway revealed a decreased frequency with the Aircast compared to the control, but the amplitude was not significantly affected. There was no tendency to shift body weight either anteriorly or posteriorly, which was similar to the finding reported during static evaluation.

In a follow-up study in 1994, Feuerbach and associates[29] found that anesthetizing the ATFL alone and in combination with the CFL did not appear to cause a decrease in proprioception of the ankle. Absolute and variable errors were diminished, however, with the Aircast, indicating that the brace may play a role in facilitating proprioception via stimulation of cutaneous receptors.

A 1994 study by Bennell and Goldie[5] concluded that optimal postural control was observed while subjects wore no ankle support and while they wore the OAPL Elastic Brace (Orthopedic Appliances Pty Ltd., Melbourne, Victoria, Australia). In contrast, postural control was compromised in the Swede-O-Universal trial.

Immobilization Versus Early Mobilization Studies

The effect of early mobilization versus immobilization following ankle injury has been clinically investigated by a few researchers.

A 1990 study conducted by Milford and Dunleavy[92] concluded that for grade I and II ankle sprains, treatment with an Aircast orthosis did not facilitate recovery from injury compared with management with conventional strapping. Individuals with a grade III sprain who wore the Aircast Walking Brace needed fewer sessions of rehabilitation (average = 6.4) and experienced fewer missed days from duty (average = 23.8) than the group managed with plaster casts.

Klein and colleagues[68] reported in 1991 that an early mobilization group wearing the Aircast demonstrated higher functional and reduced symptomology scores (46.5 points) than the immobilized, casted group (37.2 points). No difference was found radiographically between the groups with regard to talar tilt and anterior drawer prior to or following completion of the study.

A 1994 study by Eiff and associates[26] concluded that at a 10-day follow-up, an early mobilization group wearing the Aircast Air-Stirrup combined with weight-bearing gait exhibited better ROM and weight-bearing ability than a nonweight-bearing group immobilized in a posterior plaster splint. The immobilization group complained of more pain at the 3- and 6-week follow-up sessions. There was no difference between groups throughout the 1-year follow-up sessions with regard to swelling and functional abilities. Complaints of pain between the groups were significant only at the third follow-up session, where the immobilization group had more pain than the early mobilization group. Both groups returned to work full time, on average, less than 2 weeks after injury, and both groups demonstrated excellent long-term recovery.

Patient Assessment of Ankle Orthoses

Many clinical studies of ankle orthoses have incorporated the wearer's subjective comments relative to comfort, support, and effects on performance. The preference of orthosis based on the aforementioned criteria has been extremely variable among wearers, with no single brace emerging as optimal in all categories. Clinical studies are presented in accordance with the specific braces studied.

DONJOY ALP. In a 1994 study by Gross et al,[48] subjects reported the DonJoy ALP to be more comfortable than the subtalar sling, although the sling provided greater support and was more cosmetic in appearance. Many of the subjects reported discomfort during exercise while wearing both ankle supports.

AIRCAST AIR-STIRRUP AND DONJOY ALP. In a study comparing the Aircast Air-Stirrup and the DonJoy ALP orthoses, 75% of the subjects reported the Air-Stirrup to be the most comfortable brace, and 63% reported the DonJoy ALP to be more supportive.[50]

AIRCAST AIR-STIRRUP AND SWEDE-O-UNIVERSAL. In another clinical study, the Air-Stirrup was ranked highest for comfort followed by the Swede-O-Universal and the tape supports. Adhesive strapping was perceived as providing the greatest support followed by the Air-Stirrup and the Swede-O-Universal, which were equally rated. One subject complained of a pinching sensation, and two subjects developed blisters following testing with the Air-Stirrup.[51]

DONJOY ALP AIRCAST AIR-STIRRUP, AND KALLASSY. In a 1992 study by Alves and associates,[1] the Kallassy Brace was found to be the most comfortable whereas the DonJoy ALP was noted to be the most uncomfortable, with complaints of friction about the heel and cutting into the plantar aspect of the foot during plantarflexion movements. Additionally, the DonJoy ALP reportedly provided the least amount of ankle support, and the Air-Stirrup supported the most.

KALLASSY AND SWEDE-O-UNIVERSAL. Of 22 subjects who participated in a 1991 study by Burks and associates,[15] 17 reported the Swede-O-Universal Ankle Brace to be less comfortable than the Kallassy Brace or adhesive tape, which were equally comfortable. Approximately 50% of the subjects commented that the Kallassy Brace had the least detrimental effect on performance, whereas the Swede-O-Universal was felt to affect performance most negatively. Ten individuals noted that the ankle taping provided the most stability, followed by the Swede-O-Universal and the Kallassy, which were given similar ratings with respect to the amount of support.

AIRCAST AIR-STIRRUP, DONJOY ALP, AND SWEDE-O-UNIVERSAL. Greene and Wright[45] reported in 1990 that subjects preferred the DonJoy ALP for its comfort, stability, and lack of detrimental effect on performance. This orthosis was followed in preference by the Swede-O-Universal and the Aircast Air-Stirrup. Participants in a 1994 study rated the Swede-O-Universal, the Aircast Training Brace, the Aircast Sport-Stirrup, and the DonJoy ALP in terms of support, comfort, and detrimental effect on speed and quickness. In all four categories, the DonJoy ALP scored the lowest. The most supportive and the least restrictive of speed were reported to be the Swede-O-Universal and both of the Aircast braces. Overall, the Swede-O-Universal was preferred by a greater number of participants over both the Aircast Training and the Sport-Stirrup braces.[6]

ACTIVE ANKLE, AIRCAST SPORT-STIRRUP, AND MALLEOLOC. Still another study reported the Active Ankle to be the brace most preferred by wearers, followed in rank by the Sport-Stirrup and the Malleoloc, which were equally rated, and the DonJoy ALP, which was least preferred. The Active Ankle and the Sport-Stirrup were reported to have the greatest ease in application and comfort, followed by the DonJoy ALP and the Malleoloc, although these differences were not significant. With regard to stability, the Sport-Stirrup ranked higher than the Malleoloc. The Active Ankle was rated superior to the DonJoy ALP. Variable responses were given regarding functional performance for each of the orthoses.[62]

RELATED CONDITIONS OF THE ANKLE REGION

Stress Fractures

Stress fractures of the leg typically occur in individuals who are involved in activities that produce repetitive or excessive loading stresses to the tibia or fibula over a period of time. The microtrauma created by the loading stresses exceeds the bone's ability to repair itself, resulting in eventual breakdown and subsequent failure.[11]

Pathomechanics and Mechanism of Injury

Various theories regarding the pathomechanics of stress fractures have been suggested throughout the literature. As early as 1958, Devas[22] proposed that the repeated contraction of the gastrocnemius-soleus muscle complex created an "anterior bowing" of the tibia. This tibial bowing resulted in an increase in force transmitted to the posterior medial aspect of the tibia.[22] This theory for the mechanism of injury was later supported by Jackson and Bailey[60] in 1975.

Another proposed theory is that an area of increased vascularity within the tibia causes stimulation of osteoclastic resorption along the length of the haversian canal. Approximately 3 weeks following the beginning of resorption, these resorption cavities become refilled. Hyperostosis occurs with continued overuse, and a resultant fracture may occur prior to the development of sufficient callus.[63]

Stanitski[113] suggested that stress fractures occur as a result of increased and concentrated muscle forces repeatedly acting across the tibia, thereby enhancing structural loading.

The common thread in these proposed mechanisms is that all suggest repetitive stress to a specific area of bone within the tibia, stimulating a remodeling of bone in those areas and a resultant failure and microfracture of the trabeculae.[33, 41, 86, 103] As these increased stresses on the bone continue, the periosteal resorption exceeds lamellar bone formation resulting in the possibility of an associated disruption of the cortex and a subsequent stress fracture.[85]

The thinness of the cortex at the posterior medial region of the tibia, which is unsupported by cancellous bone, accounts for this site's being most commonly involved in the diagnosis of stress fractures.[60]

In addition to the pathomechanics described, nutritional deficiencies have been suggested as possibly contributing to the development of stress fractures. Inadequate nutrition may interfere with the normal osteoblastic activity necessary for bone formation.[127]

Effect of Pneumatic Compression on Stress Fracture Healing

In a study on the effect of a venous tourniquet on fracture healing, Kruse and Kelly[70] reported that the increase in venous pressure facilitated healing. It was suggested that the combination of weight bearing and a cast or cast brace promoted increased hydrostatic pressure changes in soft tissue, but also increased intramedullary blood pressure.[70, 109]

The application of a pneumatic leg brace in an animal model led to faster fracture healing than occurred with a plaster cast. The increase in hydrostatic and venous pressures causes a shifting of fluids and electrolytes from the capillary space to the interstitial fluid space. The electronegative charge that is thus created facilitates the piezoelectric effect, thereby stimulating osteoblastic activity in the bone. This bone-forming osteoblastic activity, in turn, increases the bone rate of repair.[21, 60, 70, 118]

Pneumatic leg braces also unload the tibia and fibula by stabilizing surrounding musculature, thereby reducing the anterior bowing of the tibia. By ultimately dissipating the stresses away from the fracture site, the braces permit it to heal.[22, 60, 113, 118] Additionally, the increased hydrostatic pressure within the soft tissues is believed to contribute some stability to the fracture site. Pneumatic splints used as compressive dressings following knee surgery kept effusion to a minimum compared with similar cases in which no compressive support was applied.[54] Matsen and Krugmire[88] reported that postinjury swelling was minimized by the application of 10 mm Hg of pressure applied through an airsplint.

Orthoses

The braces used in the management of stress fractures are described in Table 5–3.

TABLE 5–3
Stress Fracture Orthoses

Orthoses	Design Characteristics	Function
Aircast Air-Stirrup Leg Brace	Premolded plastic double upright lined with air cells Sizes of 20 or 40 cm in length Extends from foot to upper third of tibia	Relieves stress Promotes healing
Aircast Brace	Two plastic half shells connected with Velcro straps Four separate air bags attached to inner surface of shells One air bag over each leg surface Walking heel attached to posterior shell	Relieves stress Promotes healing

EFFECTIVENESS IN CLINICAL TRIALS. A 1987 study by Dickson and Kichline[24] reported that 13 subjects diagnosed with stress fractures were able to immediately return to sports activities after application of the Aircast Air-Stirrup Leg Brace with no detrimental effects to performance (Fig. 5–13). Eleven of the actively competing athletes were asymptomatic within 1 month. The remaining two continued to have some discomfort although not enough to interfere with continued sports participation.

Whitelaw and associates[127] observed in 1991 that all patients diagnosed with tibial stress fractures and shin splints were nontender to palpation and were able to ambulate without pain in an average of 1 week following application of an Aircast Brace (Fig. 5–14). Resumption of intensive training occurred an average of 3.7 weeks following diagnosis of injury, and preinjury competitive level was achieved an average of 5.3 weeks after Aircast Brace application.

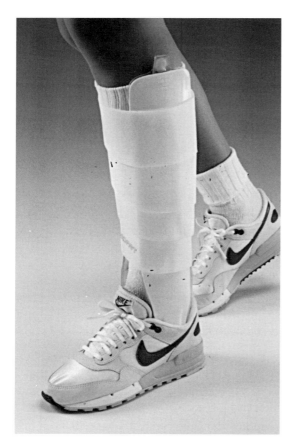

FIGURE 5–13. Aircast Air-Stirrup Leg Brace. (Courtesy of Aircast, Inc., Summit, NJ.)

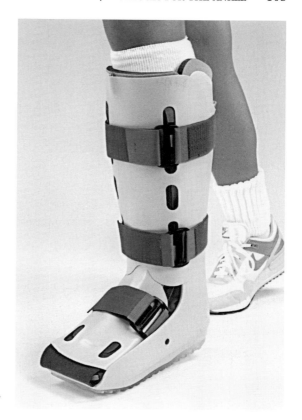

FIGURE 5–14. Aircast Brace. (Courtesy of Aircast, Inc., Summit, NJ.)

Achilles Tendinitis

Achilles tendinitis, considered to be an overuse injury, usually occurs as a result of repetitive stresses to the tendon via running and jumping activities.

Pathomechanics and Mechanism of Injury

The incidence of Achilles tendinitis has been reported to be from 6.5% to 18% among runners.[19, 69] Achilles tendinitis, Achilles tenosynovitis, and retrocalcaneal bursitis may occur from the point of insertional attachment of the Achilles tendon on the calcaneus up to 5 cm proximally on the tendon (Fig. 5–15).[73] Insertional tendinitis, which may be associated with bony protuberance of the os calcis, involves the tendon-bone interface. Noninsertional tendinitis is found immediately proximal to the calcaneal attachment, from 2 to 6 cm proximal to the calcaneus, in or around the tendon itself. In this area, the tendon internally rotates before attaching to the bone, possibly resulting in an increase in localized torque stresses.[17] The clinical findings associated with Achilles tendinitis may include diffuse pain

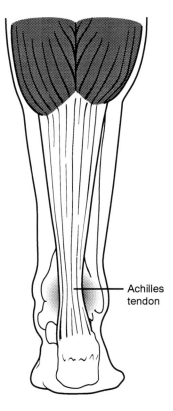

FIGURE 5–15. Site of Achilles tendinitis.

in the area of the Achilles tendon, inflammation and thickening of the peritendon, and crepitation during dorsiflexion and plantarflexion.[18]

Angiographic and isotropic studies have revealed an area of decreased vascularity in the Achilles tendon 2 to 6 cm above the calcaneal insertion.[55, 71] Lagergren and Lindholm[71] proposed that this area of diminished blood supply may predispose individuals to tendinitis within this region.

Normal stresses on the Achilles tendon range from 2000 to 7000 N.[114] Scott and Winter[110] reported that forces of 6 to 10 times a person's body weight are transmitted through the Achilles tendon during a running cycle and may result in inflammation with overuse.

Achilles tendinitis most commonly results from repetitive microtrauma but may occur with direct contact or sudden twisting injury.[7] Functional overpronation has been attributed as a cause of Achilles tendinitis.[4, 18, 61] Pronation of the foot is accompanied by tibial internal rotation, causing the Achilles tendon to be pulled medially, resulting in a bowstring effect. During the midstance phase of the gait cycle, the foot remains excessively pronated while the knee extends. Knee extension movements tend to create an external rotary force to the tibia, whereas pronation of the foot creates an internal

TABLE 5–4
Achilles Tendon Orthoses

Orthoses	Design Characteristics	Function
M-P Achilles Strap	Neoprene sleeve to cover Achilles tendon Three-dimensional triangular pad Vertical channel to accommodate tendon Counterforce bar Velcro closure	Decreases stress on tendon
Cho-Pat Achilles Strap	Tubular strap, wider anteriorly around distal calf Distal band supporting rearfoot Velcro closure	Decreases stress on tendon

rotation moment. The result of these opposing rotary forces causes excessive stress in the Achilles tendon, potentially contributing to injury.[18]

Other common causes of Achilles tendinitis include poor flexibility of the gastrocnemius-soleus muscles, improper footwear, and excessive training techniques.[17, 18]

Orthoses

The orthoses used in the treatment of Achilles tendinitis are described in Table 5–4 and are represented in Figures 5–16 and 5–17.

EFFECTIVENESS IN CLINICAL TRIALS. Two clinical studies investigated the effects of heel inserts on the management of Achilles tendinitis. In 1981 MacLellan and Vyvyan[82] concluded that all but one patient with Achilles tendinitis had a satisfactory outcome, both functionally and with regard to symptoms, after 3 months of wearing viscoelastic heel inserts. Following 3 months of wearing

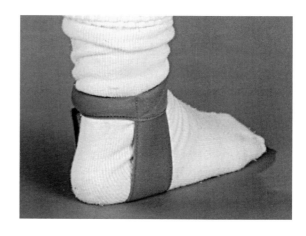

FIGURE 5–16. Cho-Pat Strap.

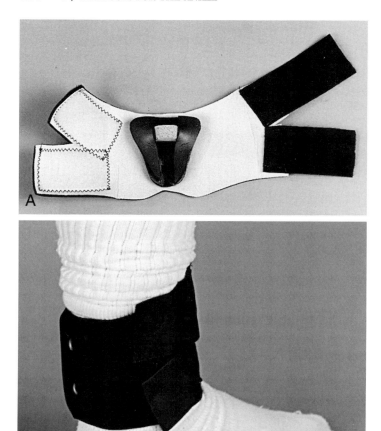

FIGURE 5–17. M-P Achilles Strap. *A*, Ready to apply. *B*, Strap in place.

inserts, only one person in the group with pain beneath the heel complained of any symptoms. Additionally, all patients with heel pain returned to full competitive sports at the end of the 3-month period. A 1984 study by Lowdon and associates[78] determined that the untreated control group demonstrated greater significant differences in the reduction of pain and swelling than the groups treated with Sorbothane heel pads and soft sponge pads of moleform (Hinders-Leslie, Ltd., London, UK). Additionally, the group with the soft sponge-rubber heel pads exhibited more significant changes in the parameters studied than did the group with the Sorbothane pads.

A 1994 study investigating the effects of the M-P Achilles Strap on eccentric plantarflexion torque concluded that no difference in peak torque occurred between braced and unbraced normal male subjects (see Fig. 5–17). However, a lower peak torque was observed in women wearing the strap than in those subjects in the unbraced trials.[93]

Plantar Fasciitis

The plantar fascia, which extends from the calcaneal tuberosity to the plantar aspect of the metatarsal heads, is subject to inflammation as a result of trauma, overuse, abnormalities in foot structure/function, and tightness.

Pathomechanics and Mechanism of Injury

Plantar fasciitis is an inflammatory reaction to microtearing within the plantar fascia.[7] One cause of plantar fasciitis is a decreased flexibility of the Achilles tendon, resulting in excessive pronation and a subsequent abnormal stretch to the plantar fascia.[90] Prolonged pronation during the stance phase of the gait cycle does not allow for normal supination to occur prior to push-off. As a result, the foot does not become a rigid lever for push-off but remains a flexible "bag of bones." The result is excessive stresses to the plantar fascia (Fig. 5–18).[97, 126]

A cavus foot may also predispose a person to this pathologic condition because of the inability to provide shock absorption and to dissipate forces.[121]

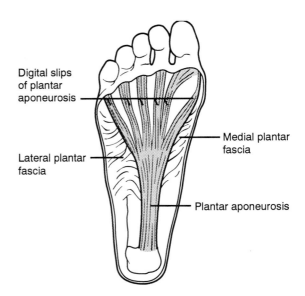

FIGURE 5–18. Site of plantar fasciitis.

TABLE 5–5
Plantar Fasciitis Orthosis

Orthosis	Design Characteristics	Function
Plantar Fasciitis Night Splint	Molded plastic footplate from calcaneus to forefoot to hold in 10 to 20 degrees of dorsiflexion Lateral and medial strut Can be disassembled for travel	Maintains plantar fascia stretch

Orthoses

The proposed rationale for orthotic intervention in plantar fasciitis is that the foot remains in a resting plantarflexed position during the night, causing the Achilles tendon and the plantar fascia to shorten. Upon arising and weight bearing, the patient forcibly stretches the plantar fascia and the Achilles tendon thereby perpetuating the inflammatory process. It is believed that the night splint, positioned in dorsiflexion, prevents this shortening of these structures and prevents reinjury upon initial weight bearing.[125] The orthosis used in the management of plantar fasciitis is described in Table 5–5.

EFFECTIVENESS IN CLINICAL TRIALS. A 1991 study by Wapner and Sharkey[125] reported that 11 subjects with pain at the insertional site of the plantar fascia became asymptomatic within 4 weeks of wearing the Plantar Fasciitis Night Splint (Orthomerica Products, Inc., Newport Beach, CA, and Orlando, FL) (Fig. 5–19).

SUMMARY

The use of orthotic intervention at the ankle is well documented throughout the literature. Researchers have concluded that the limitation of inversion-eversion ROM to within normal physiologic values can assist in the reduction of the incidence of injury and reinjury to the ankle. The restriction of excessive ankle inversion-eversion movements must be balanced by the ability of the orthosis to allow for sufficient amounts of motion so that normal, functional mechanics are not disrupted.[49, 67]

Myburgh and colleagues[94] reported that an increase in ankle ROM, although not statistically significant, was evident following exercise in unsupported ankles and that this increase in motion was a result of a "warming-up" effect of the surrounding supportive musculature. In light of this finding, the effectiveness of an ankle orthosis to restrict ankle movements following a bout of exercise becomes more critical than its ability to control the ankle at rest.

Another consideration in establishing the efficacy of an orthosis to restrict

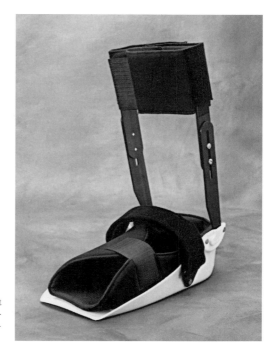

FIGURE 5–19. Plantar Fasciitis Night Splint. (Courtesy of Orthomerica Products, Inc., Newport Beach, CA, and Orlando, FL.)

ankle inversion-eversion is the structure of the talocrural joint. It has previously been discussed that the anterior portion of the talus is broader than its posterior aspect. Consequently, the ankle is more stable in a position of dorsiflexion because the anterior talus fits snugly under cover of the mortise. The unstable, plantarflexed position of the ankle is most commonly associated with ankle injuries. An orthosis prescribed for such an injury should have the ability to restrict abnormal, excessive amounts of inversion-eversion when the ankle is in a plantarflexed position.

Virtually all ankle injuries occur secondary to dynamic loading of the ankle and foot in a closed-chain situation. Studies of ankle orthoses that attempt to simulate functional ROM and weight-bearing loads are most credible when evaluating the effectiveness of an ankle support. During open-chain testing at 180 degrees per second on the Cybex 340, Gehlsen et al[40] noted the maximal combined dorsiflexion-plantarflexion ROM to be 63.5 degrees when subjects were wearing the Active Ankle Training Brace and 61.7 degrees when they were wearing the Aircast Air-Stirrup. Functional ankle ROM demands have not been as great in closed-chain activities. Milbron and Cavanaugh[91] reported only 48.2 degrees of dorsiflexion-plantarflexion motion measured electrogoniometrically during level treadmill running at 3.4 meters per second. Furthermore, Lindley and Kernozek[77] reported 29.3 and 28.6 degrees of combined dorsiflexion-plantarflexion for persons wearing the Active Ankle and the Aircast Air-Stirrup, respectively, during closed-chain testing.

The functional and performance abilities of an individual also warrant consideration in the selection of an orthosis. In addition to an ankle support providing protection from abnormal motion, it is critical that the device not have a detrimental effect on functional performance. An individual who perceives the orthosis to be a hindrance to activity will not be compliant in its use. Additionally, comfort and cosmesis play integral roles in the selection and the use of an ankle support.

There are not many specific ankle orthoses available for management of Achilles tendinitis, stress fractures of the leg, and plantar fasciitis. The available orthoses described in this chapter have been studied with respect to the effects on symptom relief and return to functional activity. Functional pronation has been identified as a common causative factor in all of these pathologic conditions, and correction of the pronation through the use of a custom foot orthosis is discussed in Chapter 6. Pathologic conditions occurring secondary to pronation could be managed with a custom foot orthosis to correct faulty biomechanics in combination with the orthoses described in this chapter to allow for an earlier return to premorbid functional, pain-free activity. Causes of other ankle and foot conditions need to be identified and corrected by the clinician to obtain long-term successful resolution of symptoms. During that process, orthotic management can be an effective adjunctive means of controlling symptoms and facilitating functional ability.

REFERENCES

1. Alves TW, Alday RV, Ketcham DL, et al: A comparison of the passive support provided by various ankle braces. J Orthop Sports Phys Ther 15:10–18, 1992.
2. Attarian DE, McCrackin HJ, DeVito DP, et al: Biomechanical characteristics of human ankle ligaments. Foot Ankle 6:54–58, 1985.
3. Balduini F, Tetzloff J: Historical perspective on injuries of the ligaments of the ankle. Clin Sports Med 1:37–53, 1982.
4. Bates BT, Osternig LR, Mason B: Foot orthotic devices to modify selected aspects of lower extremity mechanics. Am J Sports Med 7:338–342, 1979.
5. Bennell KL, Goldie PA: Differential effects of external ankle support on postural control. J Orthop Sports Phys Ther 20:287–295, 1994.
6. Beriau MR, Cox WB, Manning J: Effects of ankle braces upon agility course performance in high school athletes. J Athletic Training 29:224–230, 1994.
7. Black HM, Brand RL: Injuries of the foot and ankle. In Scott WN, Ninonson B, Nicholas JA (eds): Principles of Sports Medicine, Baltimore, Williams & Wilkins, 1984, pp 162–176.
8. Blyth CS, Mueller FO: Football injury survey. Part 1: When and where players get hurt. Physician Sportsmed 2(9):45–52, 1974.
9. Bocchinfuso C, Sitler MR, Kimura IF: Effects of two semirigid prophylactic ankle stabilizers on speed, agility, and vertical jump. J Sport Rehab 3:125–134, 1994.
10. Boruta PM, Bishop JO, Braly WG, et al: Acute lateral ankle ligament injuries: A literature review. Foot Ankle 11:107–113, 1990.
11. Brody DM: Running injuries. Clin Symp 39:2–36, 1987.

12. Brostrom L: Sprained ankles. I. Anatomic lesions in recent sprains. Acta Chir Scand 128:483–495, 1964.
13. Bunch RP, Bednarski K, Holland D, et al: Ankle joint support: A comparison of reusable lace-on braces with taping and wrapping. Physician Sportsmed 13(5):59–62, 1985.
14. Burgess PR, Wei J, Clark FJ, et al: Signaling of kinesthetic information by peripheral sensory receptors. Annu Rev Neurosci 5:171–187, 1982.
15. Burks RT, Bean BG, Marcus P, et al: Analysis of athletic performance with prophylactic ankle devices. Am J Sports Med 19:104–106, 1991.
16. Carroll MJ, Rijke AM, Perrin DH: Effect of the Swede-O-Ankle Brace or Talar tilt in subjects with unstable ankles. J Sport Rehab 2:251–267, 1993.
17. Clain MR, Baxter DE: Achilles tendinitis. Foot Ankle 13:482–487, 1992.
18. Clement DB, Taunton JE, Smart GW: Achilles tendinitis and peritendinitis: Etiology and treatment. Am J Sports Med 12:98–103, 1984.
19. Clement DB, Taunton JE, Smart GW, et al: A survey of overuse running injuries. Physician Sportsmed 9:47–58, 1981.
20. Cox JS: Surgical and nonsurgical treatment of acute ankle sprains. Clin Orthop 198:118–126, 1985.
21. Dale PA, Brook JT, Kelly PJ: Fracture healing with elevated venous pressures. ORS 35th Annual Meeting, Las Vegas, NV, February 6–8, 1989.
22. Devas MB: Stress fractures of the tibia or shin soreness. J Bone Joint Surg 40B:227, 1958.
23. Dias LS: The lateral ankle sprain: An experimental study. J Trauma 19:266–269, 1979.
24. Dickson TB, Kichline PD: Functional management of stress fractures in female athletes using a pneumatic leg brace. Am Journal Sports Med 15:86–89, 1987.
25. Distefano VJ: Anatomy and biomechanics of the ankle and foot. J Athletic Training 16:43–47, 1981.
26. Eiff MP, Smith AT, Smith GE: Early mobilization versus immobilization in the treatment of lateral ankle sprains. Am J Sports Med 22:83–88, 1994.
27. Ekstrand J, Gillquest J: Soccer injuries and their mechanisms: A prospective study. Med Sci Sports Exerc 15:267–270, 1983.
28. Feuerbach JW, Grabiner MD: Effect of the Aircast on unilateral postural control. J Orthop Sports Phys Ther 17:149–154, 1993.
29. Feuerbach JW, Grabiner MD, Koh JS, et al: Effect of an ankle orthosis and ankle ligament anesthesia on ankle joint proprioception. Am J Sports Med 22:223–229, 1994.
30. Floriana LD: Ankle injury mechanism and treatment guide. Physician Sportsmed 4:72–78, 1976.
31. Freeman MAR, Dean MRE, Hannam IWF: The etiology and prevention of functional instability of the foot. J Bone Joint Surg 47B:678–685, 1965.
32. Fumich RM, Ellison AE, Geierin GH: The measured effect of taping on combined foot and ankle motion before and after exercise. Am J Sports Med 9:165–170, 1981.
33. Furey JG, McNamee DC: Air splints for long-term management of osteogenesis imperfecta. J Bone Joint Surg 55A:645–649, 1973.
34. Garn S, Newton RA: Kinesthetic awareness in subjects with multiple ankle sprains. Phys Ther 68:1667–1671, 1988.
35. Garrick JG: The frequency of injury, mechanism of injury, and epidemiology of ankle sprains. Am J Sports Med 5:241–242, 1977.
36. Garrick JG: Ankle injuries: Frequency and mechanism of injury. J Athletic Training 10:109–111, 1975.
37. Garrick JG, Requa RK: The epidemiology of foot and ankle injuries in sports. Clin Sports Med 7:29–36, 1988.
38. Garrick JG, Requa RK: Role of external supports on prevention and treatment of ankle injuries. Med Sci Sports Exerc 5:200–203, 1973.
39. Gauffin H, Tropp H, Odenrick P: Effect of ankle disc training on postural control in patients with functional instability of the ankle joint. Int J Sports Med 9:141–144, 1988.
40. Gehlsen GM, Pearson D, Bahamonde R: Ankle joint strength, total work, and ROM: Comparison between prophylactic devices. J Natl Athletic Trainers Assoc 1:62–65, 1991.
41. Gilacli M, Milgrom C, Stein M, et al: Stress fractures and tibial bone width: A risk factor. J Bone Joint Surg 69B:326, 1987.
42. Glick JM: A study of ligamentous looseness and its relation to injury. Proc LeRoy Abbott Orthop Soc 1:34–39, 1971.
43. Greene TA, Hillman SK: Comparison of support provided by a semirigid orthosis and

adhesive ankle taping before, during, and after exercise. Am J Sports Med 18:498–506, 1990.

44. Greene TA, Roland GC: A comparative isokinetic evaluation of a functional ankle orthosis on talocalcaneal function. J Orthop Sports Phys Ther 11:245–252, 1989.
45. Greene TA, Wright CR: A comparative support evaluation of three ankle orthoses before, during, and after exercise. J Orthop Sports Phys Ther 11:453–466, 1990.
46. Gross MT: Effects of recurrent lateral ankle sprains on active and passive judgements of joint position. Phys Ther 67:1505–1509, 1987.
47. Gross MT, Ballard CL, Mears HC, et al: Comparison of Donjoy Ankle Ligament Protector and Aircast Sport-Stirrup orthoses in restricting foot and ankle motion before and after exercise. J Orthop Sports Phys Ther 16(2):60–67, 1992.
48. Gross MT, Batten AM, Lanm AL, et al: Comparison of Donjoy Ankle Ligament Protector and Subtalar Sling Ankle Taping in restricting foot and ankle motion before and after exercise. J Orthop Sports Phys Ther 19(1):33–40, 1994.
49. Gross MT, Bradshaw MK, Ventry LC, et al: Comparison of support provided by ankle taping and semirigid orthosis. J Orthop Sports Phys Ther 9(1):33–39, 1987.
50. Gross MT, Everts JR, Roberson SE, et al: Effect of Donjoy Ankle Ligament Protector and Aircast Sport-Stirrup orthoses on functional performance. J Orthop Sports Phys Ther 19:150–156, 1994.
51. Gross MT, Lapp AK, Davis J: Comparison of Swede-O-Universal Ankle Support and Aircast Sport-Stirrup orthoses and ankle tape in restricting eversion-inversion before and after exercise. J Orthop Sports Phys Ther 13(1):11–19, 1991.
52. Guise ER: Rotational ligamentous injuries to the ankle in football. Am J Sports Med 4:1, 1976.
53. Hamilton WG: Sprained ankles in ballet dancers. Foot Ankle 3:99–102, 1982.
54. Hartman JT: The use of pneumatic splint as a compression dressing. Cleve Clin Q 32:1–4, 1965.
55. Hastad K, Larsson LG, Lindholm A: Clearance of radiosodium after local deposit in the Achilles tendon. Acta Chir Scand 116:251–255, 1958–1959.
56. Hughes LY, Stetts DM: A comparison of ankle taping and a semirigid support. Physician Sportsmed 11:99–103, 1983.
57. Hutton PAN: Ankle lesions. In Jenkins DHR (ed): Ligament Injuries and Their Treatment, Baltimore, Aspen, 1985, pp 177–185.
58. Inman VT: The Joints of the Ankle, Baltimore, Williams & Wilkins, 1976.
59. Jackson DW, Ashley R, Powell J: Ankle sprains in young athletes: Relation of severity and disability. Clin Orthop 101:201–205, 1974.
60. Jackson DW, Bailey D: Shin splints in young athletes: A non-specific diagnosis. Physician Sportsmed 3:45, 1975.
61. James SL, Bates BT, Osternig LR: Injuries to runners. Am J Sports Med 6:40–50, 1978.
62. Johnson DE, Veale JR, McCarthy GJ: Comparative study of ankle support devices. J Am Podiatr Med Assoc 84:107–113, 1994.
63. Johnson LC: Morphologic analysis in pathology. In Froot HM (ed): Bone Biodynamics, Boston, Little Brown, & Co., 1964, pp 603–615.
64. Kannus P, Renstrom P: Treatment for acute tears of the lateral ligaments of the ankle. J Bone Joint Surg 73A:305–312, 1991.
65. Kaumeyer G, Malone T: Ankle injuries: Anatomical and biomechanical considerations necessary for development of an injury prevention program. J Orthop Sports Phys Ther 1:171–177, 1980.
66. Kelikian H, Kelikian AS: Disruption of the fibular collateral ligament. In Kelikian H, Kelikian AS (eds): Disorders of the Ankle, Philadelphia, W.B. Saunders Co., 1985, pp 437–496.
67. Kimura IF, Nawoczenski DA, Epler ME, et al: Effect of the Air-Stirrup in controlling ankle inversion stress. J Orthop Sports Phys Ther 9(5):190–193, 1987.
68. Klein J, Rixen D, Albring TH, et al: Functional treatment with a pneumatic ankle brace versus cast immobilization for recent ruptures of the fibular ligament in ankle. Unfallchirurg 94:99–104, 1991.
69. Krissoff WB, Ferris WD: Runners injuries. Physician Sportsmed 7(12):55–64, 1979.
70. Kruse RL, Kelly PJ: Acceleration of fracture healing distal to a venous tourniquet. J Bone Joint Surg 56A:730, 1974.

71. Lagergren C, Lindholm A: Vascular distribution in Achilles tendon—an angiographic and microangiographic study. Acta Chir Scand 116:491–495, 1958–1959.
72. Lassiter T, Malone T, Garret W: Injury to the lateral ligaments of the ankle. Orthop Clin North Am 20:629–640, 1989.
73. Leach RE, James S, Wasilewski S: Achilles tendinitis. Am J Sports Med 9:92–97, 1981.
74. Lenstrand A: Lateral lesions in sprained ankles. A clinical and roentgenological study with special reference to anterior instability of the talus. Unpublished Doctoral Dissertation, Lund, Sweden, University of Lund, 1976.
75. Leonard MH: Injuries of the lateral ligaments of the ankle. J Bone Joint Surg 31A:373–377, 1949.
76. Lindenfield TH: The differentiation and treatment of ankle sprain. Orthopedics 2:103–106, 1988.
77. Lindley TE, Kernozek TW: Taping and semirigid bracing may not affect ankle functional range of motion. J Athletic Training 30:108–112, 1995.
78. Lowdon A, Bader DL, Mowat AG: The effect of heel pads on the treatment of Achilles tendinitis: A double blind trial. Am J Sports Med 12:431–435, 1984.
79. Mack RP: Ankle injuries in athletics. J Athletic Training 10:94–95, 1975.
80. Mack KS, Douglas MS, Kum SKC, et al: Effects of Sport-Stirrup and Taping on Ankle Inversion. Unpublished Master's Thesis, Springfield, MA, Springfield College, 1994.
81. MacKean LC, Bell G, Burnham RS: Prophylactic ankle bracing vs. taping: Effects on functional performance in female basketball players. J Orthop Sports Phys Ther 22:77–81, 1995.
82. MacLellan GE, Vyvyan B: Management of pain beneath the heel and Achilles tendinitis with visco-elastic heel inserts. Br J Sports Med 15:117–121, 1981.
83. Macpherson K, Sitler M, Kimura I, et al: Effects of a semirigid and softshell prophylactic ankle stabilizer on selected performance tests among high school football players. J Orthop Sports Phys Ther 21:147–152, 1995.
84. Maehlom S, Daljord O: Acute sports injuries in Oslo: A one-year study. Br J Sports Med 18:181–185, 1984.
85. Maidment JS: The effects of ankle prophylactic devices on agility. Unpublished Master's Thesis, Springfield, MA, Springfield College, 1990.
86. Markey KL: Stress fractures. Clin Sports Med 6:405, 1987.
87. Martin M, Harter RS: Comparison of inversion restraint provided by ankle prophylactic devices before and after exercise. J Athletic Training 28:324–329, 1993.
88. Matsen FA, Krugmire R: The effect of externally applied pressure on post-fracture swelling. J Bone Joint Surg, 56A:1586–1591, 1974.
89. McCluskey GM, Blackburn TA, Lewis T: Prevention of ankle sprains. Am J Sports Med, 4:151–157, 1976.
90. McKenzie DC, Clement DB, Taunton JE: Running shoes, orthotics, and injuries. Sports Med 2:334–347, 1985.
91. Milbron MJ, Cavanaugh PR: Sagittal plane kinematics of the lower extremity during distance running. In Cavanaugh PR (ed): Biomechanics of distance running, Champaign, IL, Human Kinetics, 1990, pp 65–105.
92. Milford PI, Dunleavy PJ: A pilot trial of treatment of acute inversion sprains to the ankle by ankle supports. J Roy Nav Med Serv, 76: 97–100, 1990.
93. Morales A, Kimura I, Sitler M, et al: Effect of the Achilles tendon adhesive taping and Pro M-P Achilles Strap on eccentric plantar flexion peak torque. Unpublished Master's Thesis, Temple University, Philadelphia, PA, 1994.
94. Myburgh KH, Vaughan CH, Isaacs SK: The effects of ankle guards and taping on joint motion before, during and after a squash match. Am J Sports Med 12:441–446, 1984.
95. National Athletic Injury/Illness Reporting System, Sports Research Institute, Center for Health Aspects of Sports. Unpublished manuscript. University Park, PA, The Penn State University, 1981.
96. Nawoczenski DA, Owen MG, Ecker ML, et al: Objective evaluation of peroneal response to sudden inversion stress. J Orthop Sports Phys Ther 7:107–109, 1985.
97. Newell SG, Miller SJ: Conservative treatment of plantar fascial strain. Physician Sportsmed 5:68–73, 1977.
98. Nitz AJ, Dobner J, Kersey D: Nerve injury and grades II and III ankle sprains. Am J Sports Med 13:177–182, 1985.
99. Paris DL: The effects of the Swede-O, New Cross, and McDavid ankle braces and adhesive

ankle taping on speed, balance, agility, and vertical jump. J Athletic Training 27:253–256, 1992.

100. Paris DL, Jones D: The effect of ankle braces on inversion and eversion ranges of motion at zero and 20 degrees of plantarflexion after extended period of activity. Unpublished manuscript. Montreal, Quebec, Canada, Concordia University, 1994.

101. Paris DL, Vardaxis V, Kokkaliaris J: Ankle ranges of motion during extended activity periods while taped and braced. J Athletic Training 30:223–228, 1995.

102. Pienkowski D, McMorrow M, Shapiro R, et al: The effect of ankle stabilizers on athletic performance. Am J Sports Med 23:757–762, 1995.

103. Prather JL, Nusynowitz ML, Snody AJ, et al: Scintigraphic findings in stress fractures. J Bone Joint Surg 59A:896, 1977.

104. Rarick GL, Bigley G, Karst R: The measurable support of the ankle joint by conventional methods of taping. J Bone Joint Surg 44A:1183–1190, 1962.

105. Redford JB (ed): Orthotics Etcetera, 3rd ed, Baltimore, Williams & Wilkins, 1986.

106. Rengstrom P, Wertz M, Incavo S, et al: Strain in the lateral ligaments of the ankle. Foot Ankle 9:59–63, 1988.

107. Rovere GD, Clarke TJ, Yates CS, et al: Retrospective comparison of taping and ankle stabilizers in preventing ankle injuries. Am J Sports Med 16:228–233, 1988.

108. Sandelin J: Acute sport injuries. A clinical and epidemiological study. Unpublished Doctoral Dissertation, Helsinki, Findland, University of Helsinki, 1988.

109. Sarmiento A: A functional below-the-knee cast for tibial fractures. J Bone Joint Surg 49A:855–875, 1967.

110. Scott SH, Winter DA: Internal forces at chronic running injury sites. Med Sci Sports Exerc 22:357–369, 1990.

111. Shapiro MS, Kabo JM, Mitchell PW, et al: Ankle sprain prophylaxes: An analysis of the stabilizing effects of braces and tape. Am J Sports Med 22(1):78–82, 1994.

112. Sitler M, Ryan J, Wheeler B, et al: The efficacy of semirigid ankle stabilizers to reduce acute ankle injuries in basketball. Am J Sports Med 22:454–460, 1994.

113. Stanitski CL, McMaster JH, Scranton PE: On the nature of stress fractures. J Sports Med 6:391, 1978.

114. Staples OS: Rupture of the fibular collateral ligament of the ankle. Results of study of immediate surgical treatment. J Bone Joint Surg 57A:101, 1975.

115. Staples OS: Ligamentous injuries of the ankle joint. Clin Orthop 42:21–34, 1965.

116. Stormont DM, Mairey BF, An KN, et al: Stability of the loaded ankle. Am J Sports Med 13:295–300, 1985.

117. Stover CN: Air-Stirrup management of ankle injuries in the athlete. Am J Sports Med 13:360–365, 1980.

118. Stover CN, York JM: The Aircast/Air-Stirrup system for graduated management of lower extremity injuries. A scientific exhibit paper. San Francisco, CA, American Academy of Orthopedic Surgeons, 1979.

119. Stuessi E, Tiegermann V, Gerber H, et al: A biomechanic study of the stabilization effect of the Aircast Ankle Brace, 10th International Congress of the ISB, Umea, Sweden, June 15, 1985.

120. Surve I, Schwellness MD, Noakes T, et al: A five fold reduction in the incidence of recurrent ankle sprains on soccer players using the Sport-Stirrup Orthoses. Am J Sports Med 22:601–605, 1994.

121. Tanner SM, Harvey JS: How we manage plantar fasciitis. Physician Sportsmed 16:39–47, 1988.

122. Tropp H, Askling C, Gillquist J: Prevention of ankle sprains. Am J Sports Med 18:259–262, 1985.

123. Tropp H, Ekstrand J, Gillquist J: Stabilometry in functional instability of the ankle and its value in preventing injury. Med Sci Sports Exerc 16(1):64–66, 1984.

124. Tropp H, Odernrick P, Gillquist J: Stabilometry recordings in functional and mechanical instability of the ankle joint. Int J Sports Med 6:180–182, 1988.

125. Wapner KL, Sharkey PF: The use of night splints for treatment of recalcitrant plantar fasciitis. Foot Ankle 12:135–137, 1991.

126. Warren BL: Plantar fasciitis in runners: Treatment and prevention. Sports Med 10:338–345, 1990.

127. Whitelaw GP, Wetzler MJ, Levy AS, et al: A pneumatic leg brace for the treatment of tibial stress fractures. Clin Orthop 270:301–305, 1991.

CHAPTER 6

Orthoses for the Foot

DEBORAH A. NAWOCZENSKI

The use of foot orthoses has been accelerated by the fitness explosion over the past two decades and the rapid increase in the occurrence of overuse injuries.[33, 41, 43] Over this short span, the manufacture of foot and shoe orthoses has flourished into a $3 billion-plus industry that is expected to surpass $4 billion by 1997 according to medical and pedorthic sources.[90] Unfortunately, this growth in the orthotic industry has not been paralleled by investigative studies to support the remedial, preventive, or therapeutic value of orthotic use. Continued research in this area is necessary in order to bridge the gap between the frequency with which foot orthoses are used and the knowledge base on which their use should be founded.

This chapter focuses on the anatomic and biomechanical features of the foot that may predispose an individual to dysfunctions of the foot and/or lower extremity and that may warrant orthotic consideration. A description of foot orthotic appliances, including inserts, shoes, and shoe modifications, is presented together with a summary of the effectiveness of foot orthoses in clinical and laboratory trials.

ANATOMIC AND BIOMECHANICAL OVERVIEW OF FOOT FUNCTION

The ability of the foot to attenuate the forces of weight bearing, to accommodate to changes in terrain, and then to convert to a stable lever in preparation for propulsion approximately 500 milliseconds later requires the coordinated efforts of numerous muscles, tendons, ligaments, and bones.[17, 36, 39, 81, 88] Certain pathologic conditions or malalignment syndromes of the foot may disturb the normal biomechanical relationship of the foot and lower limb. Emerging evidence suggests a causal relationship between foot structure and activity-related musculoskeletal injuries of the hip, knee, ankle, and foot.[12, 30, 34, 46, 75, 83, 94, 103–105]

For ease of interpreting the biomechanical examination and orthotic prescription process, the foot can be divided into three functional regions: the rearfoot (or hindfoot), the midfoot, and the forefoot. The rearfoot is composed of the talus and calcaneus. The midfoot consists of the navicular, cuboid, and cuneiform bones. The forefoot includes the metatarsals and their respective phalanges. The function of the foot has also been described in terms of medial and lateral columns.[4, 16, 66] The medial column is composed of the talus, the navicular bone, the cuneiform bones, and the first three metatarsals. The primary function of the medial column is adaptive. The lateral column consists of the calcaneus, the cuboid bone, and the fourth and fifth metatarsals. These osseous components are bound together by soft tissue, with the major contributing structures being the long and short plantar ligaments. Because of its inherent stability, the lateral pillar serves as a supporting mechanism, particularly during the propulsive phase of gait.

Regardless of the anatomic delineation, the regions of the foot function as interdependent units during the stance phase of gait. Alterations in mobility and function of any region have an impact on structures both intrinsic and extrinsic to the foot. The bones of the foot and functional delineation are shown in Figure 6–1.

The diversity of approaches to the foot and ankle complex not only has led to considerable variation regarding its operation but also has resulted in considerable confusion in terminology used to describe foot motion. The motions of the ankle-foot complex can be defined operationally by motion in the sagittal, frontal, and transverse planes. Motion in the sagittal plane is described as *dorsiflexion* and *plantarflexion.* Motion in the frontal plane is known as *eversion* and *inversion.* Motion in the transverse plane is defined as *abduction* and *adduction.*[35, 89, 114] Although the motions of the foot and ankle are defined in terms of the cardinal planes, the true mechanical axes of the joints of the foot complex for the most part are *not* perpendicular to these cardinal planes but lie at some oblique orientation to these planes.[35, 39, 88, 89, 109, 114] Because motions of the foot occur perpendicular to the axis of rotation, it follows that these motions occur in planes other than the cardinal planes. The motions that occur in planes that pass through all three cardinal planes are known as *triplanar* motions.[66, 79, 88, 89, 114]

To describe triplanar motions of the foot, the terms *pronation* and *supination* are used. Pronation refers to the combined movements of abduction, dorsiflexion, and eversion. Supination refers to adduction, plantarflexion, and inversion.[79, 88, 89] The ankle, the subtalar and the midtarsal joints, and

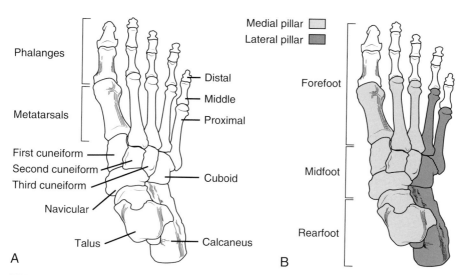

FIGURE 6–1. The anatomic *(A)* and functional *(B)* classifications of the foot. The foot can be delineated into rearfoot, midfoot, and forefoot regions. The foot has also been classified according to its functional role as a medial or lateral pillar.

the first and fifth rays have axes of motion that are oblique to the cardinal planes. Because of the axis orientation, motion at these joints can be described in terms of pronation and supination. These joints also demonstrate large variability in their axis orientation.[35, 39, 57, 89] The nonweight-bearing motions of the foot can be described in relationship to the relatively "fixed" tibia and fibula and are shown in Figure 6–2.

Deviations in foot structure purportedly result in changes in the orientation of the foot axes, which in turn lead to abnormal or compensatory movement patterns of other joints of the foot or lower-extremity kinematic chain.[75, 88, 94] Considerable attention in recent years has been directed to the subtalar joint (STJ) complex and its axis orientation. The STJ is considered to be the "keystone" to normal foot function. It plays a major role in force attenuation, in accommodation of the foot to the ground, and in the conversion of rotations between the foot/floor and lower limb during the stance phase of gait.[9, 57, 88, 89, 114] The coupling between foot inversion/eversion motion and axial rotation of the leg is determined, in part, by the orientation of the STJ axis.[19, 39, 46, 88] This axis, which indicates the magnitude and direction of rotational motion available, varies according to the structure of the foot and also varies within the foot during pronation and supination.[23, 24, 39, 57, 88, 109] This coupling between the foot and leg in weight bearing, primarily attributed to the axis orientation of the STJ, is illustrated in Figure 6–3. During weight bearing, the calcaneus is unable to accomplish all the component motions of nonweight-bearing pronation or supination on account of a combination of superincumbent body weight and frictional forces

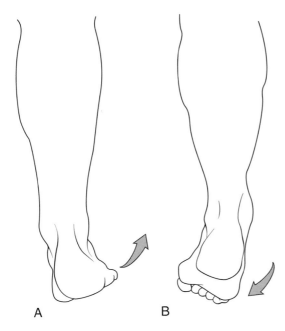

A   B

FIGURE 6–2. Triplanar, non-weight-bearing motions of the foot. Pronation of the foot includes the motions of abduction, dorsiflexion, and eversion (A). Supination includes the motions of adduction, plantarflexion, and inversion (B).

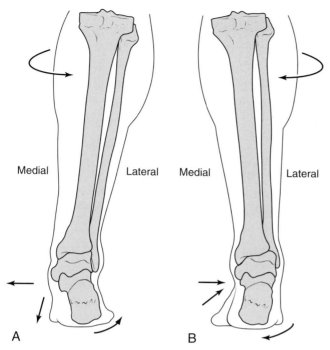

FIGURE 6-3. The coupled rotations between the foot and leg during pronation and supination in the weight-bearing limb. During pronation *(A)*, the calcaneus everts. The talus adducts and plantarflexes over the relatively fixed calcaneus. The tibia and fibula accompany talar movement and internally rotate. During supination *(B)*, the calcaneus inverts, and the talus abducts and dorsiflexes, relative to the calcaneus. The tibia and fibula accompany talar motion and externally rotate.

between the foot and the ground. The calcaneus is able to invert and evert, but other components of STJ pronation and supination occur as a result of talar movement.[52, 53, 87] By means of talar abduction/adduction and talar dorsiflexion/plantarflexion, weight-bearing STJ pronation and supination directly influence the segments and joints adjacent to it.[52, 53, 92] With weight-bearing STJ pronation, talar adduction is accompanied by medial (or internal) rotation of the tibia and fibula. Conversely, STJ supination results in talar abduction and lateral (or external) rotation of the tibia and fibula (Fig. 6-3).

This "coupling" between the weight-bearing foot and leg occurs throughout the stance period of gait as the foot pronates and supinates. The foot alternates between being a mobile, flexible adapter during weight acceptance via pronation, and a stable, rigid lever during propulsion by means of supination. Alterations in the normal coupling mechanism may lead to injuries as a result of excessive motion, inadequate motion, inappropriate sequence or timing, or a combination of these factors.

An abnormal coupling mechanism between the foot and leg has been associated with structural deformities of the foot and may lead to characteristic activity-related injuries of the hip, knee, ankle, and foot.[11, 12, 71, 75, 107] Abnormal STJ pronation not only has been linked to injuries in the foot but also has been associated with a wide range of injuries along the entire kinematic chain. These injuries include lower tibial stress fractures and shin splints,[58, 110] medial knee joint pain,[33, 54, 55, 61] retropatellar pain and knee extensor mechanism dysfunction,[15, 38, 54] chronic strain of the insertion of the gluteus maximus muscle, and greater trochanteric bursitis.[66]

An increase in activity-related injuries of the foot and lower-extremity kinematic chain also has been associated with abnormal supination. These injuries include plantar fasciitis, tibial and femoral stress fractures,[54, 58, 93] patellofemoral stress syndrome, lateral knee joint pain,[54, 62, 104] iliotibial band tendinitis,[12, 42, 88, 93] and low back pain.[113]

Foot Function in Gait

The reader is referred to Chapter 8 for an overview of the normal gait cycle, subphases, and critical events of gait. Table 6–1 highlights the kinematics of the leg and foot during the stance phase of gait. This table represents a compilation of the literature on foot function during gait and should serve as a guideline for clinical observation of gait during the biomechanical foot evaluation.[17, 40, 81, 85, 88, 114]

A review of the literature regarding foot function in gait quickly makes apparent the difficulties in attempting to study and to describe motion of the foot. The variations in foot structure, the "dynamic" and variable nature of the joint axes,[4, 35, 57, 88, 109] the triplanar motion capabilities of the joints, and the use of various models and coordinate systems to describe foot behavior present challenges to interpretation of foot function during gait.

BIOMECHANICAL EXAMINATION OF THE FOOT: A GUIDELINE FOR ORTHOTIC PRESCRIPTION

A basic understanding of the dynamic characteristics of the foot commonly begins with assessment under static conditions. The static characteristics of each foot influence its dynamic response to walking and running.[6, 85] Excellent resources that describe the lower-quarter assessment for skeletal malalignment are available.[26, 32, 112] Detailed descriptions of measurements and testing techniques are presented in these references and are recommended for the practitioner who may be unfamiliar with foot examinations. To serve as a guideline for orthotic recommendation, a lower-extremity evaluation worksheet is presented in Table 6–2. This evaluation includes assessment of stress patterns, range-of-motion assessment of the lower-extremity kinematic

TABLE 6–1
Leg and Foot Kinematics During the Stance Phase of Gait

	Weight Acceptance: Initial Contact to Loading Response (0%–12% of Gait Cycle)	
Leg and Rearfoot	*Midfoot*	*Forefoot*
Tibia rotates from a position of external rotation at heel contact to internal rotation. Ankle plantarflexes approximately 10 degrees. Calcaneus everts as STJ pronates.	MTJ joint pronation (about oblique axis) with "unlocking" of cuboid and navicular.	Forefoot contact by end of loading response. Supinated relative to midfoot and rearfoot (about longitudinal axis).

	Single Limb Support: Midstance to Terminal Stance (12%–50% of Gait Cycle)	
Leg and Rearfoot	*Midfoot*	*Forefoot*
Anterior movement of tibia. Reversal of tibial rotation from maximum internal rotation to external rotation by terminal stance. Ankle dorsiflexion to 10 degrees by end of terminal stance. STJ pronation maximum between 25% and 50% of stance. Calcaneus inverts to accompany STJ supination to neutral position by end of this period.	MTJ pronation relative to rearfoot. Osseous "locking" of calcaneocuboid joint stabilizes forefoot against rearfoot by end of this period.	Plantarflexion of medial forefoot to maintain forefoot contact by end of this phase. Osseous locking of calcaneocuboid joint in combination with ligamentous tension stabilizes forefoot on rearfoot.

	Swing Limb Advancement: Preswing (50%–62% of Gait Cycle)	
Leg and Rearfoot	*Midfoot*	*Forefoot*
Tibia external rotation reaches maximum prior to toe-off. Ankle plantarflexion to 20 degrees by end of preswing. STJ supination. Calcaneus inversion.	Midtarsal joint supination (about oblique axis) accompanies STJ supination.	Significant first ray plantarflexion at this phase. May be described as "pronation twist" of forefoot relative to midfoot.

MTJ = midtarsal joint; STJ = subtalar joint.

TABLE 6–2
Biomechanical Evaluation of the Foot: Lower-Extremity Evaluation Worksheet

Name _____   Activity (that may provoke symptoms) _____

Age _____   Shoe size _____

Sex _____   Current footwear _____

Weight _____   Orthosis wearer Y N

Height _____   Orthotic description _____

   I. **Problem (chief complaint)**

 II. **History**

III. **Objective Examination**

     A. *Posture*

     B. *Stress Patterns* (Note calluses and excessive shoe wear patterns)

        1. Feet

        2. Shoes

                                L   R   L   R

     C. *Static Measurements*

        The following static measurements can be made with the STJ in neutral and landmarks identified on leg and calcaneal segments.

1. Prone	L	R	Comments
Dorsiflexion (knee extended)			
Dorsiflexion (knee flexed)			
Plantarflexion			
Calcaneal inversion			
Calcaneal eversion			
STJ neutral (rearfoot to lower leg)			
Forefoot to rearfoot			
First ray position (N, DF, PF)*			
First ray mobility (WNL, +PF, +DF)†			

TABLE 6–2
**Biomechanical Evaluation of the Foot: Lower-Extremity
Evaluation Worksheet** *Continued*

	L	R	Comments
2. Supine/sitting/sidelying			
First ray mobility (WNL, +PF, +DF)†			
Tibial torsion			
SLR			
Hip internal rotation (note if changes with hip flexed and extended)			
Hip external rotation			
Hip flexors (opposite knee flexed)			
Leg length (note landmarks)			
Iliotibial band			

	L	R	Comments
3. Standing			
Resting calcaneal position			
Neutral calcaneal position			
Single-limb support—calcaneal position			
Tibial varum			
Q angle			
Great toe extension			

	L	R	Comments
IV. Gait Assessment			
A. *Weight Acceptance*			
Forefoot or midfoot striker			
Rearfoot position (excessive inversion/eversion)			
B. *Midstance*			
Rearfoot position			
Ankle position			
Prolonged pronation			
Early heel-off			
C. *Terminal Stance/Preswing*			
Rearfoot position			
Plantarflexion/stabilization of first ray			
V. Other Comments			

STJ = subtalar joint; SLR = straight leg raise.

*Indicates if first metatarsal is aligned with metatarsal heads 2–5 (N), or if there is a positional fault into dorsiflexion relative to metatarsal heads 2–5 (DF) or plantarflexion relative to metatarsal heads 2–5 (PF).

†Indicates if there is an equal excursion into dorsiflexion and plantarflexion from neutral (WNL) or if there is an increased range of dorsiflexion motion (+DF) or an increased range of plantarflexion motion (+PF).

Adapted from Fromherz WA: Examination. In Hunt GC (ed): Physical Therapy of the Foot and Ankle: Vol 15, CPT, New York, Churchill Livingstone, Inc. 1987, p 60.

chain in various weight-bearing positions, and assessment of the function of the foot in gait. Outcomes of this examination can be used to guide orthotic recommendations.

Examination Overview

A simple assessment of callous patterns on the plantar aspect of the foot provides invaluable information regarding the degree of shear and compressive forces during stance.[66] These patterns may indicate compensations for rearfoot or forefoot deformities. Conversely, the stress patterns may indicate the inability of the foot to compensate for structural deformities. Michaud[66] described common plantar stress patterns and the foot structures that may be associated with these patterns. These callous patterns are shown in Figure 6–4. The shoe and insert, if removable, may also indicate patterns of high stress secondary to abnormal kinematics.

The range-of-motion assessment of the lower-extremity kinematic chain takes into consideration causes of abnormal foot function that may be intrinsic, i.e., arising from within the foot and ankle, or extrinsic, i.e., originating from structures outside the foot and ankle. The gait evaluation confirms the findings of the static examination.

For relational measurements within the foot, and between the foot and tibia or fibula, the STJ frequently serves as the frame of reference to guide orthotic prescription. The neutral position of the STJ has been used as the reference point to describe positional relationships of the forefoot, midfoot, rearfoot, and lower leg in both weight-bearing and nonweight-bearing conditions.[17, 26, 87, 88] The neutral position has been defined for both palpation techniques and quantitative methods. Figure 6–5 demonstrates the palpation technique for the STJ neutral position in the nonweight-bearing condition. Using the palpation technique, the practitioner locates the medial and lateral aspects of the head of the talus at the talonavicular articulation. The neutral position is the midposition of the STJ where the talus is felt to be equally prominent at both medial and lateral aspects.[17, 20, 26, 82, 87]

A second method for determining neutral position involves quantitative goniometric measurements.[29, 88, 112] Total calcaneal inversion and eversion range of motion is measured in the nonweight-bearing position. Neutral position is obtained by inverting the rearfoot one third of the total inversion/eversion range of motion from maximum eversion. Determination of the neutral position using this technique assumes that pronation normally contributes two thirds of the total STJ motion.[87]

Disagreement exists as to the most appropriate technique for determining the STJ neutral position.[29, 32, 66] Perhaps having greater importance than the selection of technique for determination of STJ neutral position are the issues related to measurement reliability and usefulness in predicting foot function under the dynamic conditions of gait. Many of the STJ palpation measurements, when subjected to reliability testing, have resulted in only

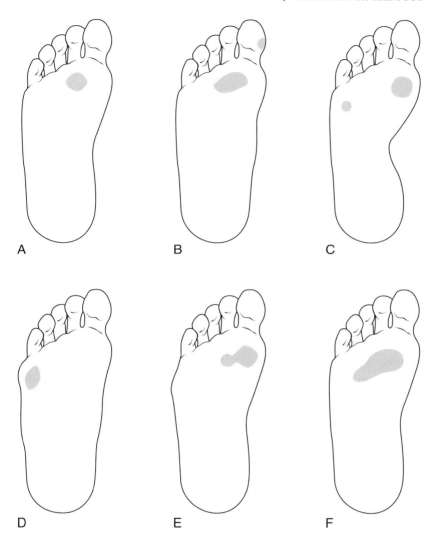

FIGURE 6–4. Plantar callous patterns provide information about the nature of the shear and compressive forces sustained during stance. The patterns may be indicative of compensated rearfoot varus *(A)*; compensated forefoot varus *(B)*; rigid plantarflexed first ray *(C)*; uncompensated rearfoot/forefoot varus *(D)*; flexible plantarflexed first ray *(E)*; or compensated equinus deformity *(F)*. (Adapted from Michaud TM: Foot Orthoses and Other Forms of Conservative Foot Care, Baltimore, Williams & Wilkins, 1993.)

poor to moderate inter- and intrarater reliability estimates.[20, 48, 82, 99] In addition to the reliability issue, there has not been strong evidence to support the relationship between static clinical measurements of the STJ and the dynamic function of the foot during gait.[34, 46, 64] Although assessment of the STJ continues to be one of the focal constituents of the biomechanical foot examination, its role in foot function may need to be reevaluated. Moreover,

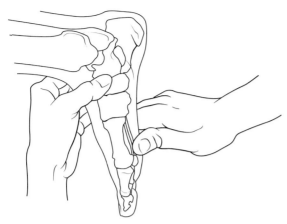

FIGURE 6-5. Palpation of the subtalar joint in neutral nonweight-bearing position. Congruency is determined by palpation of the medial and lateral aspects of the talar head at the location of the talonavicular junction.

further study is needed to enhance our understanding of the relationship between other static measurements of the biomechanical examination and the function of the foot under dynamic conditions.

STRUCTURAL AND FUNCTIONAL DEFORMITIES OF THE FOOT AMENABLE TO ORTHOTIC INTERVENTION

The biomechanical evaluation should facilitate identification of problems or deviations from the "norm" that may be improved by appropriate footwear or use of a foot orthosis. Specific goals can then be established to guide selection of appropriate inserts, shoes, or shoe modifications that will provide maximum benefit to the patient.

Structural malalignments frequently discussed in the literature may lead to hyper- or hypomobilities within the joints of the foot. Determination that a structural foot deformity exists is not necessarily a sufficient basis for prescribing treatment.[66, 107] Treatment is frequently dictated by the compensations or adjustments that may occur secondary to the deviations of another body part. These compensations most often occur at the midtarsal joint (MTJ) and STJ and result in abnormal pronation and supination.

Abnormal Pronation

Many terms are used interchangeably with the term *abnormal pronation*. These include pes planus, flatfoot or low-arched foot, valgus foot, pronated foot, and calcaneovalgus foot. The next section of this chapter addresses the deformities typically associated with acquired pes planus resulting from bony abnormalities of the ankle, the STJ or the MTJ; from trauma; or from ligamentous laxity. Abnormal pronation may also occur as a compensation for abnormalities that are extrinsic to the foot.[31, 89]

REARFOOT VARUS. This condition is defined as an intrinsic frontal plane deformity whereby the calcaneus is inverted relative to the lower leg when the foot is maintained in STJ neutral position (Fig. 6–6). Because of this excessively inverted position of the rearfoot, initial ground contact occurs along the posterolateral edge of the calcaneus. In order for the medial condyle of the calcaneus to contact the supporting surface, the STJ must pronate beyond normal, moving the calcaneus from a varus to a vertical position.[17, 32, 66, 87, 107]

FOREFOOT VARUS. In this intrinsic frontal plane deformity, the forefoot is inverted with respect to the rearfoot when the foot is maintained in STJ neutral position (Fig. 6–7). Forefoot varus may be compensated by abnormal STJ pronation, manifested by calcaneal eversion beyond vertical. This motion

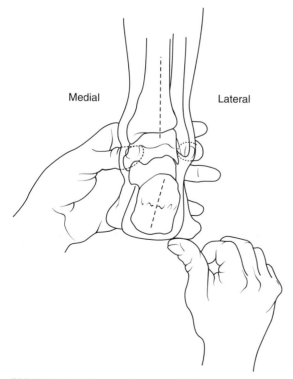

Medial   Lateral

FIGURE 6–6. The rearfoot varus deformity. The calcaneus is inverted relative to the leg when the subtalar joint is placed in neutral position.

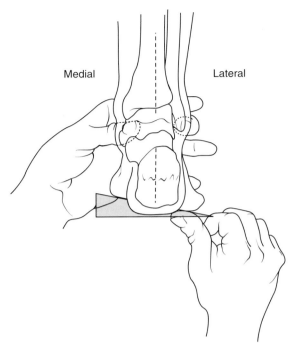

FIGURE 6–7. The forefoot varus deformity. The forefoot (metatarsal heads 2 to 5) is inverted with respect to the rearfoot when the subtalar joint is placed in neutral position.

occurs during the phase of gait when the foot should be reaching a stable position in preparation for propulsion. The deformity is frequently associated with hypermobility or dorsal shifting of the first metatarsal and inadequate stabilization of the first ray. Inadequate stabilization may predispose the metatarsophalangeal joint to problems such as hallux limitus or hallux rigidus. When there is insufficient compensation by STJ pronation, compensations may occur at the midfoot and first ray. These include midfoot abduction and excessive first ray plantarflexion, respectively.[88, 89]

ANKLE JOINT EQUINUS. This intrinsic sagittal plane deformity is defined as a lack of talocrural joint dorsiflexion when the foot is maintained in STJ neutral position. The most common cause of ankle joint equinus is limited flexibility of the gastrocnemius and soleus muscle groups.[103] Compensations for insufficient talocrural joint dorsiflexion include excessive STJ and MTJ pronation or an increase in the toe-out foot placement angle in gait.[32] Impingement exostoses may occur over time with repeated contact between the talar neck and distal tibia.[80]

STRUCTURAL OR FUNCTIONAL LEG LENGTH DISCREPANCIES. Structural leg length discrepancies are true anatomic differences in the length of the femur, tibia, or both. Functional leg length discrepancies may be described as the shortening or lengthening of a limb secondary to muscle imbalance or joint contracture.[17, 32]

ACQUIRED PES PLANUS DEFORMITIES RESULTING FROM TRAUMA AND LAXITY. Rupture of the tibialis posterior tendon is described as a cause of acquired adult pes planus foot deformity.[28, 69] The calcaneus can be described as subluxing under the talus. Ligamentous laxity is also considered an acquired pes planus deformity of the adult foot and is due to insufficient tensile strength within short and long plantar ligaments, the spring ligament, and plantar fascia.[17]

ROTATIONAL MALALIGNMENTS: TIBIAL TORSION, FEMORAL ANTEVERSION/RETRO-VERSION. These extrinsic sources of exaggerated transverse plane rotational malalignments may result in compensatory pronation.[32, 66]

Abnormal Supination

Similar to the many descriptors of the abnormally pronated foot, other terms are used interchangeably to describe the supinated foot. These terms include pes cavus and high-arched foot. The following deformities are those typically associated with cavus foot structures that lead to compensatory movements during gait.

REARFOOT VALGUS. In this intrinsic frontal plane deformity, the calcaneus is everted relative to the lower leg when the foot is maintained in the STJ neutral position (Fig. 6–8). In the uncompensated foot, this position may be maintained during the weight-bearing condition. This deformity also is present during the weight-bearing examination in cases of posterior tibialis tendon rupture.

FOREFOOT VALGUS. This intrinsic frontal plane deformity occurs when the forefoot is everted with respect to the rearfoot when the foot is maintained in STJ neutral position (Fig. 6–9). A flexible forefoot valgus may develop secondary to a rearfoot varus that is not compensated by STJ pronation. This flexibility of the forefoot allows the plantar forefoot to be brought to the ground by means of eversion about the longitudinal MTJ axis.[66, 88] A rigid forefoot valgus is compensated by abnormal STJ supination.

PLANTARFLEXED FIRST RAY DEFORMITY. In an intrinsic sagittal plane deformity of the first ray (first metatarsal, medial cuneiform), the position of the first ray is in equinus or plantarflexion (Fig. 6–10). A fixed plantarflexed first ray results in a rapid transfer of weight laterally and abnormal STJ supination.[88, 89]

It is common for any combination of forefoot or rearfoot deformities to coexist.[65, 66, 107] The manifestations of the combined foot deformities may be

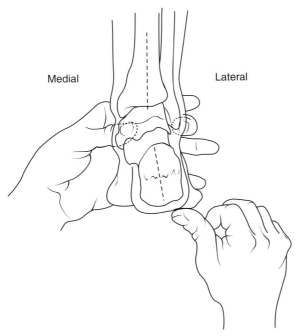

FIGURE 6–8. The rearfoot valgus deformity. The calcaneus is everted relative to the leg when the subtalar joint is placed in neutral position. In an uncompensated foot, the rearfoot remains in valgus deformity throughout stance.

different from the manifestations of the individual structural deformities. Orthotic management for combinations of malalignments can be a confusing but challenging process when one is deciding management strategies to address the deformities.

FOOT ORTHOSES

Foot orthoses are a variety of devices that are used inside the shoe to influence foot position in some way.[43] One of the primary goals of orthotic intervention is to support or "balance" the foot in order to eliminate the need for the foot to compensate for the structural deformity or malalignment.[51] Foot orthoses may also be used to provide shock absorption and to redistribute pressures throughout the plantar surface of the foot. Their use is also indicated for plantar pressure reduction through total contact fit and nonyielding relief under sites of high pressure.[43, 49, 78] Although the focus of this chapter is directed to orthotic management of structural foot deformities, the use of foot orthoses should be considered as an adjunct to treatment of lower-extremity dysfunction related to poor alignment and faulty mechan-

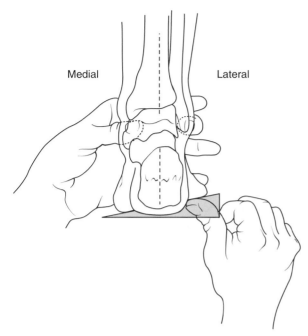

FIGURE 6-9. The forefoot valgus deformity. The forefoot (metatarsal heads 2 to 5) is everted with respect to the rearfoot when the subtalar joint is placed in neutral position.

ics. Their effectiveness is enhanced by appropriate footwear selection and selective muscle strengthening and flexibility programs when indicated.

A variety of terms are used to describe foot orthoses. These descriptions have been based on the physical properties of materials used in construction of the appliances (soft, semirigid, or rigid), the method of fabrication (molded or nonmolded), or the intended function or goal of the device (functional or accommodative). Knowledge of the physical properties of orthoses is necessary to understand the differences and indications of the various devices available on the market and their influence on function.[3] The physical characteristics of the materials frequently used in foot orthotic therapies are described in Chapter 1. The decision as to which material should be used is based on the examination findings and treatment goals.

The classification used in the following section identifies foot orthoses as soft/flexible, semirigid, or rigid. Examples of these appliances are presented in Figure 6–11.

SOFT/FLEXIBLE. Soft orthoses are used to provide cushioning, to improve shock absorption, to decrease shear forces, or to redistribute plantar pressures. These devices may also be considered accommodative.[66] Although the softer materials typically are not used when control of motion is the primary goal, they may be used in combination with other materials for

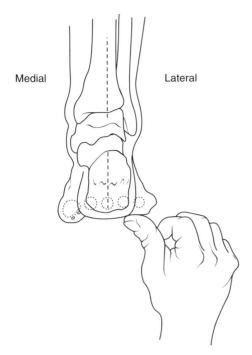

Medial

Lateral

FIGURE 6–10. Plantarflexed first ray position. The first metatarsal is plantarflexed relative to metatarsal heads 2 to 5.

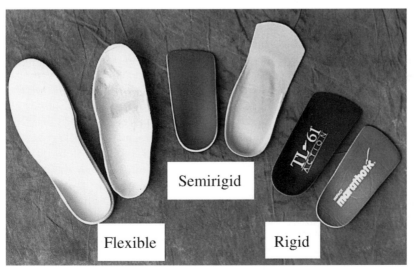

Semirigid

Flexible

Rigid

FIGURE 6–11. Three classifications of orthoses. (TL-61 and Marathotic courtesy of PAL Health Technologies, Inc., Pekin, IL.)

control of mild biomechanical imbalances.[51, 66] Soft insoles are also useful as a temporary appliance, in combination with various posting, to determine whether a permanent insole is indicated.

Low-temperature polyethylene foams currently used for orthosis construction include Plastazote (Apex Foot Products, South Hackensack, NJ), Pelite (Active International, Hillside, NJ), and Aliplast (Alimed, Dedham, MA). The different densities of these materials lend themselves to different purposes. Other soft materials include ethylene vinyl acetate (EVA) and the polyurethane materials Poron (Acor Orthopaedic, Inc., Cleveland, OH) and PPT (The Langer Biomechanics Group, Inc., Deer Park, NY). The properties of these materials make them ideal as forefoot extensions on more rigid orthotic appliances, top covers, and fillers for orthoses.[3, 49, 50] Because of their compressibility, soft insoles have a limited life span and require frequent replacement to maintain their intended purpose.

SEMIRIGID. As the name implies, semirigid insoles provide some measure of flexibility and shock absorption; however, they are more commonly used to control or to balance the malaligned foot.[51] This is accomplished through use of semirigid graphite laminates and thermoplastic materials such as polypropylene and polyethylene.[66] The durability of the prescribed semirigid device is dictated by the anticipated demands of its usage and the type of problem for which the insert is prescribed. The semirigid appliance may be a good choice when the goal is to offer some control of abnormal pronation or supination but still to provide some measure of shock absorption and pressure distribution.

RIGID. Similar to the semirigid devices, rigid insoles are used when the primary concern is to control abnormal motion. Rigid orthoses are most often made of acrylic plastics or an acrylic plastic and carbon fiber-mesh composite.[3, 96] Some providers of rigid orthoses have suggested that the rigid insole may reduce the shock-attenuation and energy-absorbing movements of the foot and may cause foot discomfort. A compromise may be the addition of a soft cover to the rigid shell, in combination with footwear that provides a good shock-absorbing outersole design (Fig. 6–12).

Fabrication of Foot Orthoses

Insoles can be nonmolded or molded. The soft insoles are typically nonmolded and can be made quickly with a minimum of materials and fabrication skill. A template of an individual's foot and shoe can be made and posting added to the inferior surface of the insole where needed. Figure 6–13 provides an example of a soft insole with options for posting at the forefoot, midfoot, or rearfoot. The temporary insoles provide the clinician with an opportunity to try different posting options and to gain feedback on their effectiveness prior to the definitive prescription.

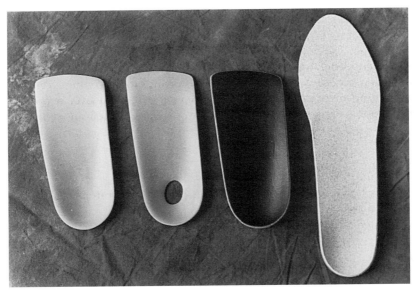

FIGURE 6-12. Modifications of a rigid design. Depending on its intended purpose, the finished orthosis can have different design features that include (from left to right) rigidity to the level of the metatarsal heads, heel relief, and partial and full covers of various densities.

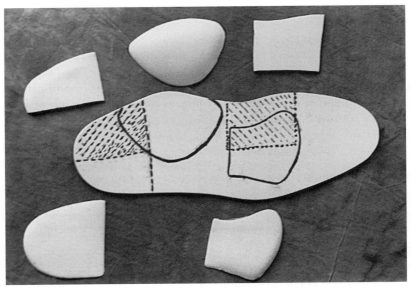

FIGURE 6-13. A temporary insole allows various posting options and provides an excellent source of evaluation and feedback prior to the definitive prescription.

Molded insoles are required for cases in which control, balance or pressure distribution, and relief are indicated. These goals can be accomplished through direct or indirect techniques. With direct molding techniques, the insole is formed under the weight-bearing foot during the molding process. The insole then can be posted or relieved according to the patient's needs. Indirect molding means that the orthotic device is formed over a positive mold of the foot. The positive mold is made from a cast of the foot frequently taken in a nonweight-bearing position, with the STJ held in neutral and the MTJ stabilized against the rearfoot. The thermoplastic materials used for the semirigid or rigid insole designs then can be formed over the mold. Because of the skill and equipment required to handle the high-temperature materials, the negative cast is frequently sent to an orthotic laboratory for fabrication of the insole.

For a detailed description of the techniques for fabrication of the foot orthoses, the reader is referred to information previously presented in the literature.[19, 66]

Achievement of Balance Through Posting

To achieve balance of a malaligned foot, additional material is added at selected locations on the plantar aspect of the insole. This additional material is called a *post*. The post is a wedge that can be used on the medial or lateral side of the insole and that is intended to support or to control movement, primarily in the frontal plane.[19] Through this buildup, the ground is essentially brought up to the weight-bearing plantar surface of the foot, thereby limiting or controlling excessive movement. Theoretically, the posts should allow the foot to function about a neutral position, rather than at the extremes of its motion capabilities.

Modifications to the insole can be made via intrinsic or extrinsic posting. Using extrinsic posting, wedges are added to the exterior surface of an orthotic insole shell (Fig. 6–14). If intrinsic posting is used, modifications are made to the shape of the positive cast impression so that the insole shell itself is able to control the deformity. Both intrinsic and extrinsic modifications can be incorporated into one insole. Figure 6–15 illustrates an example

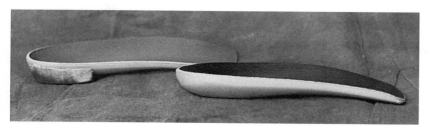

FIGURE 6–14. Foot orthoses can be posted either extrinsically (left) or intrinsically (right) at rearfoot or forefoot locations.

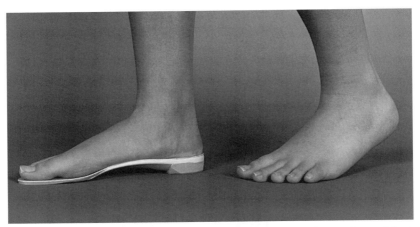

FIGURE 6–15. Example of an orthosis posted extrinsically at the rearfoot and intrinsically at the forefoot for a subject demonstrating excessive pronation during stance secondary to a forefoot varus deformity.

of an extrinsic rearfoot post and an intrinsic forefoot post for an individual with a forefoot and rearfoot varus deformity compensated by abnormal STJ and MTJ pronation.

The amount of correction incorporated into the posting of the orthoses depends on the degree of deformity, the patient's response to the posting, and the constraints of a shoe. The posting material adds bulk to the insole and frequently requires that the shoe have adequate space or depth. Changes in heel height also need to be considered with the addition of extrinsic rearfoot posts. Figure 6–16 demonstrates changes in rearfoot position and heel height with posted rearfoot orthoses for an individual with excessive pronation.

The decision as to the exact number of degrees that an orthotic shell should be posted is still controversial. Findings from clinical experience primarily have led to the recommended posting values for rearfoot and forefoot posts.[18, 19, 21, 66, 89] These values vary between posting an amount equal to the deformity to posting between 60% and 100% of the deformity. Approximately 1 mm of correction is used for every degree of deformity. Root et al[89] recommend that an orthotic device should control but not eliminate motion from heel contact to foot-flat position. As long as the normal STJ pronation is allowed to occur during the contact period, the maximum amount of recommended rearfoot posting is approximately 5 to 6 degrees.[18, 66, 88] The maximum amount of correction tolerated in the forefoot post that can fit comfortably in a shoe is approximately 8 degrees.[18, 66] Reports of clinical studies that have examined the effect of forefoot posts on STJ pronation have used corrections ranging between 60% and 100% of the deformity.[18, 21, 22] In cases where a forefoot deformity exceeds 10 degrees, combined posting of forefoot and rearfoot has been

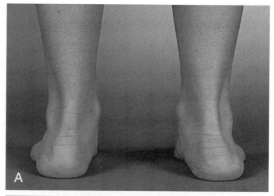

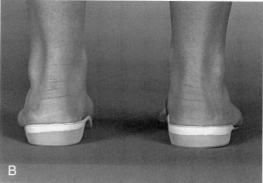

FIGURE 6–16. *A*, Excessive calcaneal eversion associated with subtalar joint pronation in a subject with a significant forefoot varus deformity. *B*, Foot orthoses were posted extrinsically in the rearfoot. The posts may increase heel height and may need to be accommodated with appropriate footwear.

suggested such that 60% of the deformity is accommodated in the forefoot post and 50% in the rearfoot post.[18, 19, 21, 22]

Additional Orthotic Considerations

HEEL LIFTS/CUPS. Heel lifts provide sagittal plane correction for ankle joint equinus and leg length discrepancy. The choice of a shock-absorbing material such as Viscolas (Chattanooga Corporation, Chattanooga, TN) or PPT for a heel lift may be effective in decreasing impact forces that may lead to retropatellar pain and stress fractures.[67] Figure 6–17 demonstrates a heel lift that also provides shock-absorbing capabilities. In some cases, heel lifts also have been an effective form of treatment for Achilles tendinitis.[66] Heel lifts may aggravate painful forefoot problems such as metatarsalgia and plantar fasciitis as weight is shifted toward the metatarsal heads. Their benefit in reducing the tendency for compensatory motions at the STJ and MTJ is debatable.

ARCH SUPPORTS. The use of arch supports to control excessive pronation may be helpful in reducing symptoms in some patients. Investigators have suggested that there may be some forefoot or rearfoot posting provided by

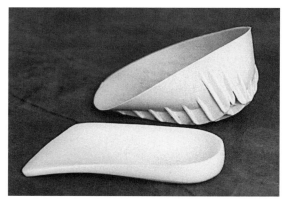

FIGURE 6–17. Heel lifts and cups may be used for ankle joint equinus and leg length discrepancies. They may also provide some shock absorption for painful heel syndromes.

the addition of an arch support, particularly if the arch thickness extends close to the metatarsal heads[5] or the calcaneus. In this case, the arch support provides some control of forefoot (or rearfoot) varus similar to that offered by a biomechanical orthosis posted for a forefoot or rearfoot varus deformity.

Reinforcement of the medial longitudinal arch of an orthosis with either PPT or cork has been suggested for the high-impact user.[66] This reinforcement would be added to the orthosis that is already posted in the rearfoot or forefoot.

ORTHOTIC "EXTRAS." Orthotic devices can be further modified by various additional components. These include top covers and horseshoe pads for redistribution of pressures away from painful lesions such as plantar warts or an accessory navicular or in cases of discrete calcaneal pain. Metatarsal pads are another option used to redistribute pressure away from the painful (and sensate) metatarsal heads by supporting the distal metatarsal shafts. These pads are available in various shapes and sizes and may be effective in temporary relief of painful interdigital neuromas, plantar keratoses, and plantar warts. They are usually fit on an individualized basis and can be easily assessed at numerous locations in the foot[37] (Fig. 6–18).

Foot orthoses should also conform to the heel height and pitch of the shoe. High-heel shoes with little room to spare for an insole can be challenging to fit. Any additional material in these shoes may cause the foot to slip out the back of the shoe or may constrict the forefoot. For this reason, thin materials such as carbon graphites, fiberglass, or composites are popular choices for fabrication of women's dress shoe orthoses (Fig. 6–19).

Orthoses also may need to be modified to accommodate the biomechanical demands associated with a specific sport. The requirements of distance running versus sprinting versus race-walking demand different control features in each of the orthoses.[7, 8, 74, 101] The requirements of running that

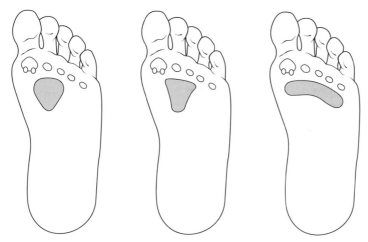

FIGURE 6-18. Examples of different shapes of metatarsal pads used to redistribute pressures away from the metatarsal head.

need to be considered in the orthotic prescription are fairly straightforward when compared with the requirements for asymmetric activities such as golf or edge sports such as skating and skiing. The golf swing requires pronation of one foot while the other foot remains stabilized throughout the swing.[111] Edge sports such as skating and skiing need the boot/foot interaction taken into consideration when foot orthoses are incorporated for the control of abnormal pronation.[58, 59]

Ballet dancing presents one of the most difficult challenges to orthotic management for foot-related problems. Orthotic laboratories are now working specifically with dancing injuries in fabricating orthoses that provide forefoot posting within a flexible or semirigid thermoplastic shell. This shell may be covered by suede or PPT and is held in place with an elastic band and a thong. Miller and colleagues[68] describe a modified ballet shoe/orthosis

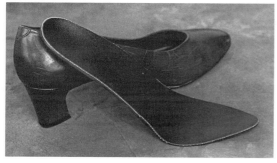

FIGURE 6-19. Foot orthoses fabricated from thinner materials such as carbon graphite, fiberglass, or composites have improved options for women wearing high heels.

combination that was able to redistribute pressures away from the frequently overworked and injured first and second metatarsal heads.

PATIENT-RELATED FACTORS RELEVANT TO THE ORTHOTIC PRESCRIPTION

In addition to understanding the properties of the materials used in orthotic construction (see Chap. 1), the practitioner must appreciate the equally important patient-related factors that play a critical role in the success of the orthotic prescription. The patient's *diagnosis* is the starting point in determining which type of material and which orthotic design are most appropriate. A patient who has diabetes and a neuropathic foot may be best served by an accommodative, total-contact insert to facilitate greater pressure distribution.[43] In the neuropathic foot that has ulcerated, a rigid relief orthosis[78] may be effective in preventing reulceration after an ulcer has healed. Patients with inflammatory arthritis who complain of foot pain exacerbated by joint motion may have relief if the foot is supported by an orthotic device constructed of more rigid or dense material. The goal of this orthosis is to offer greater stability to the foot.[3] Changes associated with feet of the older adult, including atrophy of plantar fat pads, require consideration for soft orthoses or soft top covers for the semirigid or rigid shell designs.[3]

The *weight* of the patient is important to consider when prescribing orthoses because the appliance must sustain increased forces in heavier patients. For heavier individuals (or those engaged in high-impact activities), there may be more rapid deformation of materials, resulting in bottoming out of softer materials or fatigue fracture of the orthosis itself. To prevent bottoming out, the strength of the material used in the orthosis may need to be increased (see Chap. 1). When soft insoles are prescribed for improved pressure distribution, patients should be issued extra insoles to use in their shoes on a rotation basis.[47] For similar reasons, the material of the shell of the orthoses should be matched to the demands for control of excessive motion and the *level of activity* of the individual. For high-impact activities, the orthosis needs to be durable enough to resist vertical forces on impact without undergoing fatigue fracture, rapid deformation, or bottoming out.

Cost is equally relevant in the orthotic prescription. Frequently, good footwear is the solution to many foot problems originating intrinsically or externally. In many cases, it may be the only treatment required for relief of symptoms. Before permanent orthoses are prescribed, temporary orthoses with options for modifications (see Fig. 6–13) or selective strapping techniques, such as those described in Chapter 7, should be tested. These methods are cost-effective and provide excellent feedback for assessing the potential benefit of a more permanent orthosis.

Finally, the outcome of therapy depends on the shoe and orthosis combination. The orthoses are only as effective as the shoes in which they are worn. Heel counters and outersole, midsole, and insole designs can be used to maximize the benefits of orthotic prescription. The components of footwear are discussed at the end of this chapter.

EFFECTIVENESS OF FOOT ORTHOSES IN CLINICAL TRIALS

Relief of pain and the ability to return to previous levels of activity are major considerations in determining the success of orthotic therapy.[2, 14, 18, 33] In numerous reports of recreational athletes who experienced lower-extremity symptoms that included knee pain, plantar fasciitis, posterior tibial syndrome, shin splints, or iliotibial band tendinitis, at least 75% reported marked improvement with orthotic use.[2, 14, 33] Simkin and colleagues[93] also found semirigid orthotic devices to be effective in reducing the incidence of stress-related fractures in military recruits having different foot arch structures. The incidence of femoral stress fractures was significantly reduced with orthotic use for feet with high arches, and the incidence of metatarsal fractures was reduced among feet with low arches.

Changes in Kinematic Parameters

In addition to subjective changes reported with their use, orthoses have significantly modified selected aspects of lower-extremity kinematic behavior during stance. The majority of investigations have assessed the effects of orthoses on kinematic parameters associated with abnormal pronation. Specifically, the frontal plane components of STJ motion, calcaneal inversion and eversion have been evaluated using motion analysis techniques. Two-dimensional (2D) motion analysis has been the most commonly used method to study the frontal plane angle changes between the lower leg and shoe, or between the shoe and the floor with orthotic use. Although the findings of the kinematic investigations are not always in agreement, 2D studies have demonstrated changes in rearfoot motion parameters with orthotic use that include a reduction in maximum pronation (as measured by calcaneal eversion),[2, 60, 86, 98, 106] maximum pronation velocity,[2, 77, 98] time to maximum pronation,[2, 98] and total rearfoot movement.[2, 77] Studies that reported similar findings for one variable, however, did not always report comparable results for another variable.

Reasons for the inconsistencies in findings among the 2D investigations may be attributed to design variability between, and even within, investigations. Differences in the material used for the orthoses, the magnitude and location of the posting on the orthotic insole, testing on overground versus treadmill surfaces, self-selected versus predetermined walking and running test speeds, and variations in footwear all potentially influence the outcomes of the study and preclude comparative and conclusive findings. Explicit sample description is also of considerable importance when comparing the effects of foot orthoses on kinematic responses, especially considering the inherent structural variability of each person's foot in small sample-sized studies. Confounding the issue of sample selection are the lack of clinically reliable, quantitative measurements of foot and lower-extremity angular relationships.[13, 20, 82, 99]

One of the most frequently reported measurements of effectiveness is the magnitude of calcaneal eversion controlled by the orthosis. The changes in the magnitude of maximum calcaneal eversion demonstrated with orthotic use have varied from 1 degree to 2.5 degrees[7, 86, 98] to a maximum of 4 degrees in two studies.[5, 77] These changes in frontal plane calcaneal motion have been shown with the use of semirigid and rigid orthotic designs.

Some investigators have considered a reduction in maximum pronation velocity to be a significant factor related to pain relief with orthotic use. Smith et al[98] and Novick and Kelley[77] demonstrated a decrease in angular velocity measures of the rearfoot relative to the lower leg in both running and walking studies, respectively. These findings, however, were not supported by Rodgers and LeVeau,[86] who assessed the effect of semirigid appliances on foot function in runners and found no differences in maximum pronation velocity. Discrepancies in the findings among these investigators have been attributed to differences in footwear, in testing speed, and in test surface.

In light of the increased use of motion analysis systems in the clinical environment, the limitations of 2D analysis need to be considered when studying the effect of orthotic devices on rotations of the lower kinematic chain. The angles projected onto the film plane of the camera are subjected to increasing error as the abduction or toe-out angle of the foot increases.[1] Projection errors have approached 30% on angular rotations generated from 2D analysis during running.[1, 100] During walking, distortions associated with segmental rotations out of the film plane have been maximum between 0% and 8% and after 60% of the stance period, when compared with three-dimensional (3D) data.[10] These findings have clinical implications for the assessment of orthotic effectiveness using 2D analysis techniques.

In addition to the issues associated with projection errors of 2D analysis, investigators have shown that assessment of calcaneal inversion/eversion alone may not necessarily be the best predictor of the function and orientation of the STJ.[1, 24, 53, 100] Both cadaver and human motion studies have demonstrated that calcaneal abduction/adduction when combined with inversion/eversion provides a better indicator of STJ function than single-plane analysis alone.[1, 23, 24] Analysis of the combined rotations also provides an indication of lower-limb rotation due to the direct coupling between the talus and tibia/fibula.[52, 53, 92] More recently, investigations of foot function using 3D analysis techniques have provided increased understanding of the effect of orthoses on rotational patterns of the lower limb.

One of the earlier 3D investigations of the effect of semirigid orthoses in runners with compensatory pronation was carried out by Taunton et al[106] using a triplanar goniometer to monitor the combined talocrural/subtalar joint motion and associated knee motion. The investigators found a significant decrease in the total eversion that occurred during stance between orthotic and nonorthotic conditions. In a related study using a triplanar goniometer, Smart and Robinson[97] also found that use of the orthoses reduced talocrural/subtalar motion but increased knee abduction motion during the stance period of running. The authors postulated that the reduction of frontal plane motion at the talocrural/subtalar joint necessitated a transfer of motion to more proximal structures.

Eng and Pierrynowski[22] assessed the effect of soft foot orthoses on 3D lower-extremity kinematics in 10 female subjects with patellofemoral pain during treadmill walking and running. In addition to patellofemoral pain, these subjects had clinical foot measurements of forefoot varus or calcaneal valgus. The authors assessed the changes using medially posted orthotic devices during different phases of the stance period. Minimal reductions in frontal and transverse plane motions (1 to 3 degrees) were found at the talocrural/subtalar joint during walking and running with the soft orthoses. The orthoses also reduced knee motion in the frontal plane during the initial contact and midstance phases of walking (less than 1 degree), but increased the frontal plane knee motion during these same phases of running by a similar magnitude. The authors suggested that altered loading of the patellofemoral joints, reflected by changes in transverse and frontal plane rotations, may provide one reason for reduction in pain with orthoses.[21, 22]

Nawoczenski et al[71] examined the effect of semirigid foot orthoses on 3D kinematics of the leg and rearfoot in two groups of runners (n = 20) with radiographically distinct foot structures. These groups presented clinically with pes planus or pes cavus foot types. All the subjects wore similar running sport sandals that allowed for direct visualization of rearfoot motion during running. The results of the kinematic analysis showed a significant orthotic effect for tibial internal rotation for both groups for the period between heel contact and maximum pronation. An overall mean decrease of 2 degrees in this variable represented an average 31% decrease in the total amount of tibial axial rotation over the nonorthotic condition in subjects with pes planus foot structures. In subjects with cavus foot structures, this finding represented a reduction of 22% in tibial internal rotation when compared with the nonorthotic condition. Subjects in this investigation with cavus foot types also responded favorably to semirigid orthotic intervention.

Another variable of interest in the assessment of foot orthoses and their effect on kinematic behavior is the material used in fabrication of the orthosis. Few comparative studies have been done. In one 2D study, Smith and colleagues[98] compared soft and semirigid orthoses with a shoe-only condition in a group of runners. These authors reported a significant reduction in maximum calcaneal eversion using semirigid orthoses compared with a shoe-only condition. Both soft and semirigid orthoses were equally effective in controlling maximum calcaneal eversion velocity.

Brown et al[5] compared the effects of an arch support, a semirigid orthotic device, and shoes alone on 2D rearfoot kinematics during walking. The authors assessed 24 subjects with forefoot varus deformity and directly visualized rearfoot movement by using a transparent heel counter in the shoe. These investigators found no significant reductions in maximum pronation, calcaneal eversion, or total pronation with either the arch support or the semirigid orthosis when compared with the shoes-only condition.

In addition to the materials used for fabrication, the location of posting materials on the insole has been assessed in some kinematic studies. Novick and Kelley[77] and Sims[95] found that orthoses posted in both the forefoot and the rearfoot showed reductions in rearfoot-to-leg rotations compared with shoes alone. Johanson et al[44] examined the effect of three different posting methods on controlling frontal plane motion in subjects with significant forefoot varus deformities. The subjects were assessed during walking using a nonorthotic control and four different test conditions: nonposted orthotic shells; orthosis posted in the forefoot only; orthosis posted in the rearfoot only; and orthoses posted in both the forefoot and the rearfoot. All posted devices offered some control of frontal plane motion over the nonorthotic condition. Combined rearfoot and forefoot posts and rearfoot posts alone demonstrated the most control of frontal plane eversion in this study, although the magnitude of mean differences between the orthotic conditions was approximately 1 degree.

Changes in Electromyographic Response

Changes in stability of the foot associated with abnormal pronation or supination may be accompanied by alterations in muscle activity, resulting in muscle fatigue and overuse syndromes. Few investigations have examined the effect of orthotic devices on electromyographic (EMG) changes during gait. In one walking study, Tomaro and Burdett[108] studied 10 subjects with abnormal pronation who were treated with sport orthoses. Their findings showed an increase in the duration of EMG activity of the tibialis anterior muscle with orthosis use. No changes were found in mean EMG activity of the tibialis anterior, gastrocnemius, or peroneus longus. The authors proposed that the increased duration of the tibialis anterior EMG activity may be related to the decrease in STJ velocity found in previous studies because the tibialis anterior functions to control forefoot loading during stance.

In another study, investigators examined the effect of semirigid orthoses on EMG changes of the tibialis anterior, medial gastrocnemius, vastus medialis, vastus lateralis, and lateral hamstring in 12 subjects with abnormal pronation during treadmill running.[72] The results of this investigation showed a highly individualized and variable response to orthosis use. A significant decrease in lateral hamstring mean EMG activity was found with orthosis use. This finding may be consistent with the kinematic changes associated with a reduction in tibial internal rotation for individuals with planus foot structures.[71] The authors suggest that the requirement for lateral hamstring activity to control tibial internal rotation may be reduced if the orthoses can attenuate excessive tibial motion. Although not significant, trends toward increased mean EMG activity were found in the tibialis anterior and medial gastrocnemius.

FOOTWEAR

Although the types of shoe inserts previously described are effective in balancing or in correcting mechanical abnormalities in the foot, they are rarely successful without the correct footwear. Appropriate footwear is as important as the correct design and fabrication of the orthotic appliance in the prescription process. In many cases, proper footwear may be the only recommendation needed for successful management of patient problems related to musculoskeletal alignment. Conversely, a poorly designed or recommended shoe may serve as an extrinsic source of musculoskeletal problems.

Despite the fact that participants in the fitness explosion of the past 20 years have experienced their share of musculoskeletal problems,[55, 56, 61, 102] there has been a favorable impact on footwear design characteristics to meet the needs of the user. Advances in technology of materials combined with greater options for stability and motion control have benefited not only the population of runners, but the patient populations having a variety of foot disorders as well. The following section details anatomic features of the shoe that are important components of the prescription process.

Components of the Shoe

Shoes are designed to provide a combination of flexibility, stability, and motion control. These goals are accomplished through use of assorted design features that include shoe lasts, heel counters, lacing systems, and different midsole and outersole materials.[25, 27, 45, 63, 74, 76, 101] These design features can be broadly grouped into upper and lower components. The upper components of a shoe include the vamp, the quarter, the throat, and the toe box. The lower components are the outersole, the shank, and the heel. The components of the shoe are illustrated in Figure 6–20.

THE UPPER COMPONENTS. The *vamp* extends from the instep anteriorly and covers the forefoot and toes. The vamp is joined to the *quarters*, which make up the sides and back of the upper shoe. The *throat* is defined by the line

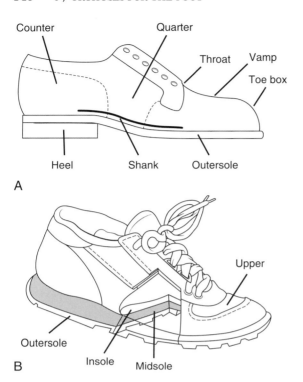

FIGURE 6–20. Components of the standard oxford-style shoe *(A)* and the athletic shoe *(B)*.

that connects the rear part of the vamp and the front part of the quarter. The throat determines the maximum foot girth permitted by the shoe. Two styles typically found in an oxford-style shoe describe the attachment of the quarter to the vamp. These styles are termed *Blucher* and *Bal*. In the Blucher style, the quarter panels are placed on top of the vamp, and the front edges are not sewn together. The Blucher style accommodates a broader foot (Fig. 6–21). In the Bal style, the front edges of the quarter panels on each side of the shoe are stitched together and are covered by the back edge of the vamp.

The *toe box* refers to the part of the shoe that covers the toes. The height and width of the toe box are determined by the shape of the last used to construct the shoe. Certain shoes offer extra depth in the toe box to accommodate deformities of the feet such as claw toes and hammer toes.

The heel *counter* is a component of the quarter that stabilizes the rearfoot in the shoe and retains the shape of the posterior portion of the shoe.[27, 63] Because of the increased pronation that occurs with running, manufacturers of footwear have enhanced rearfoot stability through various modifications of the heel counter. These include reinforcement with additional leather or plastic or by extension of the sides of the midsole superiorly to support the inferior aspect of the counter.[63] The heel counter should be firm and closely

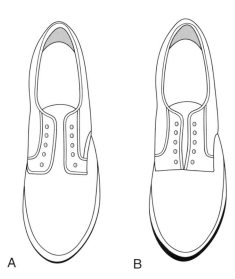

FIGURE 6–21. The Blucher *(A)* and Bal *(B)* style oxford shoes.

A   B

contoured to the patient's calcaneus in order to stabilize the rearfoot and to maintain the calcaneal fat pad.[66]

THE LOWER COMPONENTS. The *outersole* is the material between the plantar surface of the foot and the ground. The outersole should be durable and flexible (in most cases) and should provide traction. Changes in outersole geometry have influenced foot kinematics. Rigid rocker and curved outersole designs have alleviated metatarsal head pressures by eliminating the bending of the shoe at the toebreak[70, 91] (Fig. 6–22). The toe of the shoe is curved upward, which shortens the functional length of the shoe while allowing the metatarsal heads to move through a lessened range of motion during propulsion.[66] The location of the takeoff point of the rocker sole may effectively reduce the lever arm of ground-reaction forces on the ankle

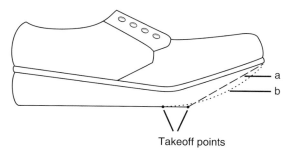

Takeoff points

FIGURE 6–22. Rocker (a) and curved or roller-outersole design (b). The takeoff or pivot point is located at or proximal to the metatarsal heads. The toe of the shoe is curved upward, which allows the metatarsals to move through less range of motion during propulsion.

joint and may decrease the magnitude of force required from the Achilles tendon to plantarflex the ankle.[27] These design features may aid in the management of Achilles tendinitis, plantar fasciitis, metatarsalgia, or hallux limitus or rigidus.[66, 84]

The *shank* of the shoe refers to the area that lies between the heel and the metatarsal heads. The purpose of the shank is to provide rigidity to the midsection of the shoe and to prevent the front of the shoe from twisting on the rear portion.[63, 84] In athletic footwear, a midsole wedge is used in place of a shank or shank/heel combination. The density of the midsole and the extent of the heel flare modify subtalar motion.[25, 27, 45, 101] The alteration in motion is brought about by a change in the effective lever arm of the ground-reaction forces at initial contact (Fig. 6–23). Because of the nature of their compressibility, softer and more flexible shoes have smaller lever arms, which, in turn, result in reduced joint torques and a decrease in the rate of pronation.[101] A shoe with a soft midsole slows the rate of pronation but also allows a greater amount of total pronation.[25, 27, 101] Shoe manufacturers have tried to address the issues of controlling the rate as well as the magnitude of pronation by combining a softer lateral midsole with a firmer medial midsole.[27, 66] The lateral side of this dual-density midsole is soft to decrease the lever arm of ground-reaction forces at initial contact and to reduce the initial velocity of pronation while firmer material on the medial side protects against excessive pronation.

The *heel* of a shoe also can be modified to effect changes in foot motion. Nigg and Morlock[74] found that a lateral heel flare increased the length of the lever arm between the STJ axis and the ground (see Fig. 6–23). This flare produced an increase in both the magnitude and the rate of STJ pronation. Although considered beneficial in certain cases of an uncompensated rearfoot varus,[63] a shoe with a lateral flare may actually cause an increase in pronation-related complaints.[27]

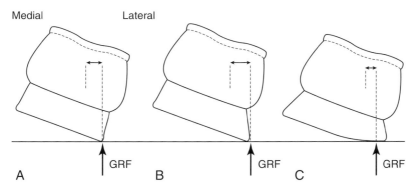

FIGURE 6–23. Both the density of the midsole material and the degree of the lateral heel flare affect the magnitude and rate of pronation during the loading response of gait. GRF = ground-reaction force.

A negative posterior heel flare (Fig. 6–24*A*) may be used to reduce the range and velocity of ankle plantarflexion between initial contact and loading response.[66] This reduction is achieved by means of a shorter lever arm between the ground-reaction forces and ankle joint axis. Conversely, a longer posterior flare (Fig. 6–24*B*) can increase the lever arm of ground-reaction forces on the ankle joint, requiring increased effort from the anterior compartment muscles and potentially giving rise to anterior shin splints.[27]

Shoe Construction

THE LAST. The *last* refers to the foot-shaped, wooden or high-density polyethylene mold over which the components of a shoe are molded. Shoes can be either straight- or curved-lasted. A straight-lasted shoe is well aligned in the forefoot and rearfoot, whereas a curved-lasted shoe is angled medially at the forefoot (Fig. 6–25). There have been various recommendations regarding the use of a straight- versus a curved-lasted shoe for different foot types,[32, 63, 66] for the most part unsubstantiated by clinical studies. Fuller's[27]

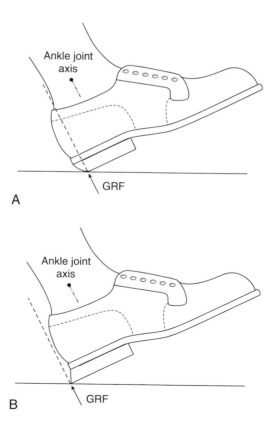

FIGURE 6–24. A posterior flare can alter the location of the ground-reaction force (GRF) vector relative to the ankle joint and can influence the plantarflexion response at initial contact.

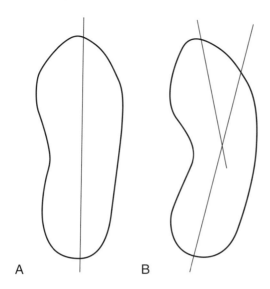

A   B

FIGURE 6–25. A straight-lasted
shoe is well aligned in the forefoot
and rearfoot *(A)*. A curved-lasted
shoe is angled medially at the forefoot *(B)*.

suggestion that the shape of the last be, most importantly, the same shape
as the foot seems to be the most practical recommendation.

Various methods are used in shoe construction to attach the upper
component to the lower component of the shoe. Shoes may be board-lasted,
slip-lasted, or combination-lasted (Fig. 6–26). A board-lasted shoe has a hard,
fibrous board on its inner surface that provides stability and that may be
beneficial in cases of excessive pronation.[32, 66] The stiffness of the board,

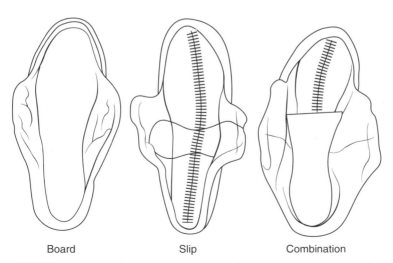

Board   Slip   Combination

FIGURE 6–26. Board-, slip-, and combination-lasted features provide varying degrees of stiffness and flexibility to the construction of the shoe.

however, may be contraindicated in cases of Achilles tendon problems.[66] The slip-lasted shoe has no insole board. It is lighter, more flexible, and roomier in the toe box than the board-lasted design. The combination-lasted shoe has features of both the board- and the slip-lasted designs. Stability is provided in the board-lasted rearfoot and midfoot, whereas flexibility is maintained in the slip-lasted forefoot. The features of stability as well as flexibility make the combination-lasted shoe a popular choice.

A combination of the footwear features previously presented has been recommended for musculoskeletal problems associated with feet that excessively pronate or supinate during stance.[25, 32, 62, 63, 73] For the hypermobile, planus, or excessively pronated foot, footwear characteristics include board- or combination-lasted designs; a firm heel counter that is reinforced on the medial aspect of the shoe; and a high-density or reinforced midsole on the medial side of the shoe. Shoe characteristics that may prove helpful in the management of the hypomobile, cavus, or excessively supinated foot include a slip-lasted design; a firm heel counter; and heel or midsole material that allows attenuation of ground-reaction forces.

Whereas certain shoe features may be more appropriate for one type of foot-related problem over another, the choice of footwear should meet the user's needs.

SUMMARY

Advances in motion analysis technology have provided increased options for studying foot function and the effect of foot orthoses and shoe designs on foot and lower-extremity movement. The variability in foot structure, orthotic designs, shoe components, and testing conditions has made comparative studies of orthotic efficacy challenging. Many aspects of orthotic intervention still need further exploration. For example, although orthoses are prescribed for compensations of both supination and pronation, most investigative studies have addressed their effectiveness in cases of excessive pronation. Likewise, our understanding of kinematic changes associated with orthotic use has been generated primarily through investigations that have been limited to assessment of rearfoot and leg rotations only. This limited view of foot function has been necessitated by the difficulty encountered in modeling the small bones of the midfoot and forefoot and in working within the constraints of current motion analysis technology. Innovations in laboratory analysis techniques will continue to broaden our comprehension of the coupling nature of forefoot, midfoot, rearfoot, and leg rotations and the impact of foot orthoses on these rotations.

The analysis of footwear takes three components into consideration: the person, the shoe, and the supporting surface. Fitness footwear offers excellent options to accommodate various patient diagnoses and various foot structures. The shoes serve as the foundation for effective orthotic intervention and should be the first consideration in the management of foot-related musculoskeletal problems.

REFERENCES

1. Areblad M, Nigg B, Ekstrand J, et al: Three-dimensional measurement of rearfoot motion during running. J Biomech 23:933–940, 1990.
2. Bates B, Osternig L, Mason B, et al: Foot orthotic devices to modify selected aspects of lower extremity mechanics. Am J Sports Med 7:338–342, 1979.
3. Berenter RW, Kosai DK: Various types of orthoses used in podiatry. Clin Podiatr Med Surg 11:219–229, 1994.
4. Bojsen-Moller F: Anatomy of the forefoot, normal and pathologic. Clin Orthop Rel Res 142:10–18, 1979.
5. Brown GP, Donatelli R, Catlin PA, et al: The effect of two types of foot orthoses on rearfoot mechanics. J Orthop Sports Phys Ther 21:258–267, 1995.
6. Cavanagh PR: The biomechanics of lower extremity action on distance running. Foot Ankle 7:197–217, 1987.
7. Clarke TE, Frederick E, Hamill C: The effects of shoe design parameters on rearfoot control in running. Med Sci Sports Exerc 15:376–381, 1983.
8. Clarke T, Frederick E, Hamill C: The study of rearfoot movement in running. In Friederick EC (ed): Sports Shoes and Playing Surfaces, Champaign, IL, Human Kinetics, 1984, pp 166–187.
9. Close J, Inman V, Poor P, et al: The function of the subtalar joint. Clin Orthop Rel Res 50:159–177, 1967.
10. Cornwall MW, McPoil TG: Comparison of 2-dimensional and 3-dimensional rearfoot motion during walking. Clin Biomech 10:36–40, 1995.
11. Cowan DN, Jones BH, Robinson JR: Medial longitudinal arch and risk of training associated injury. Med Sci Sports Exerc 21:260 (abstract), 1989.
12. Cowan DN, Jones BH, Robinson JR: Foot morphologic characteristics and risk of exercise-related injury. Arch Fam Med 2:773–777, 1993.
13. Cowan DN, Jones BH, Robinson JR, et al: Consistency of visual assessments of arch height among clinicians. Foot Ankle 15:213–217, 1994.
14. D'Ambrosia R: Orthotic devices in running injuries. Clin Sports Med 4:611–618, 1985.
15. D'Amico JC, Rubin M: The influence of foot orthoses on the quadriceps angle. J Am Podiatr Assoc 76:337–339, 1989.
16. DiGiovanni J, Smith S: Normal biomechanics of the adult rearfoot—A radiographic analysis. J Am Podiatr Assoc 66:812–824, 1976.
17. Donatelli RA: Abnormal biomechanics. In Donatelli RA (ed): The Biomechanics of the Foot and Ankle, Philadelphia, F.A. Davis Co., 1990, pp 34–72.
18. Donatelli RA, Hurlbert C, Conaway D, et al: Biomechanical foot orthotics: A retrospective study. J Orthop Sports Phys Ther 10:205–212, 1988.
19. Donatelli RA, Wooden M: Biomechanical orthotics. In Donatelli R (ed): The Biomechanics of the Foot and Ankle, Philadelphia, F.A. Davis Co., 1990, pp 28, 193–216.
20. Elveru RA, Rothstein JM, Lamb RL: Goniometric reliability in a clinical setting: Subtalar and ankle joint measurements. Phys Ther 68:672–677, 1988.
21. Eng JJ, Pierrynowski MR: Evaluation of soft foot orthotics in the treatment of patellofemoral pain syndrome. Phys Ther 73:62–69, 1993.
22. Eng JJ, Pierrynowski MR: The effect of soft foot orthotics on three-dimensional lower limb kinematics during walking and running. Phys Ther 74:836–844, 1994.
23. Engsberg JR, Andrews JG: Kinematic analysis of the talocalcaneal/talocrural joint during running support. Med Sci Sports Exerc 19:275–284, 1987.
24. Engsberg J, Grimston S, Wackwitz J: Predicting talocalcaneal joint orientations from talocalcaneal/talocrural joint orientations. J Orthop Res 6:749–757, 1988.
25. Frederick E: Kinematically-mediated effects of sport shoe design: A review. J Sports Sci 4:169–184, 1986.

26. Fromherz WA: Examination. In Hunt GC (ed): Physical Therapy of the Foot and Ankle: Vol 15, CPT, New York, Churchill Livingstone, Inc., 1987, pp 59–90.
27. Fuller EA: A review of the biomechanics of shoes. Clin Podiatr Med Surg 11:241–258, 1994.
28. Funk DA, Cass JC, Johnson JA: Acquired adult flatfoot secondary to posterior tibial tendon pathology. J Bone Joint Surg 68A:95–98, 1986.
29. Garbalosa JC, McClure MH, Catlin PA, et al: The frontal plane relationship of the forefoot to the rearfoot in an asymptomatic population. J Orthop Sports Phys Ther 20:200–206, 1994.
30. Giladi M, Milgrom C, Stein M, et al: The low arch, a protective factor in stress fractures—a prospective study of 295 military recruits. Orthop Rev 14:709–712, 1985.
31. Gould N: Evaluation of hyperpronation and pes planus in adults. Clin Orthop Rel Res 181:37–45, 1983.
32. Gross MT: Lower quarter screening for skeletal malalignment—suggestions for orthotics and shoewear. J Orthop Sports Phys Ther 21:389–405, 1995.
33. Gross M, Davlin L, Evanski M: Effectiveness of orthotic shoe inserts in the long-distance runner. Am J Sports Med 19:409–412, 1991.
34. Hamill J, Bates B, Knutzen K, et al: Relationship between selected static and dynamic lower extremity measures. Clin Biomech 4:217–225, 1989.
35. Hicks J: The mechanics of the foot. I. The joints. J Anat 87:345–357, 1953.
36. Hollinshead W, Rosse C: Textbook of Anatomy, Philadelphia, Harper & Row Publishers, Inc., 1985.
37. Holmes GB, Timmerman L: A quantitative assessment of the effect of metatarsal pads on plantar pressures. Foot Ankle 11:141–145, 1990.
38. Huberti HH, Hayes WC: Patellofemoral contact pressures. J Bone Joint Surg 64A:715–724, 1984.
39. Inman V: The Joints of the Ankle, Baltimore, Williams & Wilkins, 1976, pp 35–43.
40. Inman V, Rolston H, Todd F: Human Walking, Baltimore, Williams & Wilkins, 1981.
41. James S, Bates B, Osternig L: Injuries to runners. Am J Sports Med 6:40–50, 1978.
42. James S, Jones D: Biomechanical aspects of distance running injuries. In Cavanagh P (ed): Biomechanics of Distance Running, Champaign, IL, Human Kinetics, 1990, pp 249–269.
43. Janisse DJ: Indications and prescriptions for orthoses in sports. Orthop Clin North Am 25:95–107, 1994.
44. Johanson MA, Donatelli R, Wooden MJ, et al: Effects of three different posting methods on controlling abnormal subtalar joint pronation. Phys Ther 74:149–161, 1994.
45. Jorgensen: Body load in heel-strike running: The effect of a firm heel counter. Am J Sports Med 18:177–181, 1990.
46. Kernozek T, Richard M: Foot placement angle and arch type: Effect on rearfoot motion. Arch Phys Med Rehabil 71:988–991, 1990.
47. Kuncir EJ, Wirta RW, Golbranson FL: Load-bearing characteristics of polyethylene foam: An examination of structural and compressive properties. J Rehabil Res Dev 27:229–238, 1990.
48. Lattanza L, Gray G, Kantner R: Closed versus open kinematic chain measurements of subtalar joint eversion: Implications for clinical practice. J Orthop Sports Phys Ther 9:310–314, 1988.
49. Leber C, Evanski P: A comparison of shoe insole materials in plantar pressure relief. Prosthet Orthot Int 10:135–138, 1986.
50. Lewis G, Tan T, Shide YS, et al: Characterization of the performance of shoe insert materials. J Am Podiatr Med Assoc 81:418–424, 1991.
51. Lockard MA: Foot orthoses. Phys Ther 68:1866–1873, 1988.
52. Lundberg A, Svensson O, Bylund C, et al: Kinematics of the ankle/foot complex—Part 2: Pronation and supination. Foot Ankle 9:248–253, 1989.
53. Lundberg A, Svensson I, Bylund C, et al: Kinematics of the ankle/foot complex—Part 3: Influence of leg rotation. Foot Ankle 9:304–309, 1989.
54. Lutter L: Foot-related knee problems in the long distance runner. Foot Ankle 1:112–116, 1980.
55. Lysholm J, Wiklander J: Injuries in runners. Am J Sports Med 15:168–171, 1987.
56. Mann RA: Biomechanics of running. In American Academy of Orthopaedic Surgeons Symposium on the Foot and Leg in Running Sports, St. Louis, C.V. Mosby Co., 1982, pp 30–44.
57. Manter J: Movements of subtalar and transverse tarsal joints. Anat Rec 80:397–410, 1941.

58. Matheson GO, Clement DB, McKenzie DC: Stress fractures in athletes. A study of 320 cases. Am J Sports Med 15:46–58, 1987.
59. Matheson GO, Macintyre JG: Lower leg varum alignment in skiing: Relationship to foot pain and suboptimal performance. Physician Sportsmed 15:9, 1987.
60. McCulloch M, Brunt D, Vander Linden D: The effect of foot orthotics and gait velocity on lower limb kinematics and temporal events of stance. J Orthop Sports Phys Ther 17:2–10, 1993.
61. McKeag D, Dolan C: Overuse syndromes of the lower extremity. Physician Sportsmed 17:108–123, 1989.
62. McKenzie D, Clement D, Taunton J: Running shoes, orthotics, and injuries. Sports Med 2:334–347, 1985.
63. McPoil TG: Footwear. Phys Ther 68:1857–1865, 1988.
64. McPoil TG, Cornwall MW: The relationship between subtalar joint neutral position and rearfoot motion during walking. Foot Ankle 15:141–145, 1994.
65. McPoil TG, Knecht HG, Schuit D: A survey of foot types in normal females between the ages of 18 and 30 years. J Orthop Sports Phys Ther 9:406–409, 1988.
66. Michaud TM: Foot Orthoses and Other Forms of Conservative Foot Care, Baltimore, Williams & Wilkins, 1993, pp 61, 64–65, 186.
67. Milgrom C, Giladi M, Kashton H, et al: A prospective study of the effect of a shock-absorbing orthotic device on the incidence of stress fractures in military recruits. Foot Ankle 6:101, 1985.
68. Miller CD, Paulos LE, Parker RD, et al: The ballet technique shoe: A preliminary study of eleven differently modified ballet technique shoes using force and pressure plates. Foot Ankle 11:97, 1990.
69. Mueller TJ: Acquired flatfoot secondary to tibialis posterior dysfunction: Biomechanical aspects. J Foot Surg 30:2, 1991.
70. Nawoczenski DA, Birke JA, Coleman WC: The effect of rocker-sole design on plantar forefoot pressures. J Am Podiatr Med Assoc 78:455–460, 1988.
71. Nawoczenski DA, Cook TM, Saltzman CL: The effect of foot orthotics on three-dimensional kinematics of the leg and rearfoot during running. J Orthop Sports Phys Ther 21:317–327, 1995.
72. Nawoczenski DA, Ludewig PM: The effects of balanced foot orthotics on EMG activity of selected lower extremity musculature during running. Phys Ther 73:S101 (abstract), 1993.
73. Nigg B, Bahlsen A, Denoth J, et al: Factors influencing kinetic and kinematic variables in running. In Nigg B (ed): Biomechanics of Running Shoes, Champaign, Il, Human Kinetics, 1986, pp 139–159.
74. Nigg B, Morlock M: The influence of lateral heel flare of running shoes on pronation and impact forces. Med Sci Sports Exerc 19:294–302, 1987.
75. Nigg B, Nauchbaeur W, Cole G: Effects of arch height of the foot on angular motion of the lower extremities in running. J Biomech 26:909–916, 1993.
76. Nigg B, Segesser B: Biomechanical and orthopedic concepts in sport shoe construction. Med Sci Sports Exerc 24:595–602, 1992.
77. Novick A, Kelley D: Position and movement changes of the foot with orthotic intervention during the loading response of gait. J Orthop Sports Phys Ther 11:301–312, 1990.
78. Novick A, Stone J, Birke JA, et al: Reduction of plantar pressure with the rigid relief orthosis. J Am Podiatr Med Assoc 83:115–122, 1993.
79. Oatis CA: Biomechanics of the foot and ankle under static conditions. Phys Ther 68:1815–1821, 1988.
80. O'Donoghue DH: Impingement exostoses of the talus and tibia. J Bone Joint Surg 39:835–852, 1957.
81. Perry J: Anatomy and biomechanics of the hindfoot. Clin Orthop Rel Res 177:9–15, 1983.
82. Picciano AM, Rowlands MS, Worrell T: Reliability of open and closed kinetic chain subtalar joint neutral positions and navicular drop test. J Orthop Sports Phys Ther 18:553–558, 1993.
83. Radin EL, King HY, Riegger C, et al: Relationship between lower limb dynamics and knee joint pain. J Orthopedic Res 9:398–405, 1991.
84. Reed JK, Theriot S: Orthotic devices, shoes and modifications. In Hunt GC (ed): Physical Therapy of the Foot and Ankle: Vol 15, CPT, New York, Churchill Livingstone, Inc., 1987, pp 285–313.
85. Rodgers MM: Dynamic foot biomechanics. J Orthop Sports Phys Ther 21:306–316, 1995.

86. Rodgers MM, LeVeau B: Effectiveness of foot orthotic devices used to modify pronation in runners. J Orthop Sports Phys Ther 4:86–90, 1982.
87. Root MC, Orien WP, Weed JH: Biomechanical examination of the foot. Vol I. Los Angeles, Clinical Biomechanics Corp., 1977.
88. Root MC, Orien WP, Weed JH: Normal and abnormal function of the foot. Vol II. Los Angeles, Clinical Biomechanics Corp., 1977, pp 29–33.
89. Root MC, Weed JH, Sgarlato T, et al: Axis of motion of the subtalar joint. J Am Podiatr Assoc 56:149–155, 1966.
90. Rossi WA: Orthotics: The miracle cure-all? Footwear News May 8, 1995, p 22.
91. Schaff PS, Cavanagh PR: Shoes for the insensitive foot: The effect of a "rocker bottom" shoe modification on plantar forefoot pressures. Foot Ankle 11:129–140, 1990.
92. Siegler S, Chen J, Schneck C: The three dimensional kinematics and flexibility characteristics of the human ankle and subtalar joints. Part I: Kinematics. J Biomech Eng 110:364–373, 1988.
93. Simkin A, Leicher I, Giladi M, et al: Combined effect of foot arch structure and an orthotic device on stress fractures. Foot Ankle 10:25–29, 1989.
94. Simkin A, Leichter I: Role of the calcaneal inclination in the energy storage capacity of the human foot—a biomechanical model. Med Biol Eng Comput 28:149–152, 1990.
95. Sims DS: The effect of a balanced foot orthosis on muscle function and foot pronation in compensated forefoot varus. Thesis. Iowa City, The University of Iowa, 1983.
96. Sims DS, Cavanagh PR: Selected foot mechanics related to prescription of foot orthotics. In Jahss MH (ed): Disorders of the Foot, Philadelphia, W. B. Saunders Co., 1990, pp 469–483.
97. Smart G, Robinson G: Triplanar electrogoniometer analysis of running gait. In Winter DA, Norman R, Hayes H, et al (eds): Biomechanics I-B, Champaign, Il, Human Kinetics, pp 144–148, 1985.
98. Smith L, Clarke T, Hamill C, et al: The effects of soft and semi-rigid orthoses upon rearfoot movement in running. J Am Podiatr Med Assoc 76:227–233, 1986.
99. Smith-Oricchio K, Harris B: Interrater reliability of subtalar neutral, calcaneal inversion and eversion. J Orthop Sports Phys Ther 12:10–15, 1990.
100. Soutas-Little R, Beavis G, Verstraete M, et al: Analysis of foot motion during running using a joint co-ordinate system. Med Sci Sports Exerc 19:285–293, 1987.
101. Stacoff A, Kalin X, Stussi E: The effects of shoes on the torsion and rearfoot motion in running. Med Sci Sports Exerc 23:482–490, 1991.
102. Stanish W: Overuse injuries in athletes: A perspective. Med Sci Sports Exerc 16:1–7, 1984.
103. Subotnick SI: Equinus deformity as it affects the forefoot. J Am Podiatr Med Assoc 61:423–426, 1971.
104. Subotnick SI: The cavus foot. Physician Sportsmed 8:53–55, 1980.
105. Subotnick SI: The flat foot. Physician Sportsmed 9:85–91, 1981.
106. Taunton J, Clement D, Smart G, et al: A triplanar electrogoniometer investigation of running mechanics in runners with compensatory overpronation. Can J Appl Sports Sci 10:104–115, 1985.
107. Tiberio D: The effect of excessive subtalar joint pronation on patellofemoral mechanics: A theoretical model. J Orthop Sports Phys Ther 9:160–165, 1987.
108. Tomaro J, Burdett RG: The effects of foot orthotics on the EMG activity of selected leg muscles during gait. J Orthop Sports Phys Ther 18:532–536, 1993.
109. Van Langelaan E: Relative talotibial movements and relative tarsal movements. Acta Orthop Scand, 54:135–265, 1983.
110. Viitasalo J, Kvist M: Some biomechanical aspects of the foot and ankle in athletes with and without shin splints. Am J Sports Med 11:125–130, 1983.
111. Williams KR, Cavanagh PR: The mechanics of foot action during the golf swing and implications for shoe design. Med Sci Sports Exerc 15:247, 1983.
112. Wooden MJ: Biomechanical evaluation for functional orthotics. In Donatelli RA (ed): The Biomechanics of the Foot and Ankle, Philadelphia, F.A. Davis Co., 1990, pp 168–183.
113. Wosk J, Voloshin AS: Low back pain: Conservative treatment with artificial shock absorbers. Arch Phys Med Rehabil 66:145–148, 1985.
114. Wright DG, Desai SM, Henderson WH: Action of the subtalar and ankle joint complex during the stance phase of walking. J Bone Joint Surg 46A:361–382, 1964.

CHAPTER 7

Protective Padding and Adhesive Strapping

KATHRYN P. HEMSLEY

Supportive wrapping and bandaging techniques have been used by generations of athletically active individuals. Depictions of ancient Greeks preparing for sports activity by applying these supports to their limbs can readily be found.[6] As time-honored a tradition as these techniques have been, there is little clinical research to confirm or to deny their efficacy. Despite the relative dearth of clinical research, adhesive strapping and protective padding techniques are broadly accepted as an empirically proven adjunct to orthopaedic health care.

PRINCIPLES IN APPLICATION OF MATERIALS

Adhesive strapping and protective padding techniques may be used within the context of a rehabilitation program that is formulated from a specific diagnosis and comprehensive evaluation. The rationales for their use include management of the initial inflammatory process through immobilization, compression, and support of the involved structures and prevention of further soft tissue damage. When properly employed with the appropriate materials, strapping and padding provide a custom fit to stabilize the affected area externally while allowing the limb sufficient mobility for functional activity. Therefore, these techniques must be tailored to the individual's needs, with adjustments made as necessary throughout the clinical course.

The effectiveness of these procedures is the subject of numerous studies that are reviewed as each technique is presented in this chapter. The angle of tape application relative to the axes of motion of the joint(s) involved, the variations in the sequence of the procedures chosen for application, and the type of materials used and their adherence to the skin all can affect the extent to which the area is ultimately supported.[9] Additionally, the overall efficacy of adhesive strapping and protective padding techniques is contingent on a number of general principles underlying all the specific applications.

Positioning the joint and maintaining the desired joint position are crucial to the success of proper tape application. An understanding of the pathomechanics is integral to identifying the optimal joint position needed to avoid creating deleterious forces that could exacerbate the injury. For example, limitation of repetitive hyperextension and valgus stress to the metatarsophalangeal joint of the great toe in a patient with turf toe is necessary to protect against additional trauma. In this instance, a position of protection would be a relatively parallel alignment of the metatarsophalangeal joint with respect to the longitudinal axes of both the hallux and the metatarsal segments.

The strength of support required to maintain the desired joint position is predicated on the degree of soft tissue injury, the stage of healing, and the forces to which the injured area may be subjected. Different taping materials afford varying grades of support. The four criteria on which tape is graded are its tensile strength, the number of vertical and horizontal threads per square inch, its compositional content (cotton or synthetic fiber percentage and bleached or unbleached treatment in its manufacturing process), and its adherence mass.[9] Greater strength is found in tape with a high thread count (150 threads/square inch) that is unbleached and uncolored. Folding the tape edges also improves its strength. Another factor related to the strength of support is the variety of expansion afforded by the different densities of elastic tape currently manufactured. The degree of elasticity can be manipulated as the material is applied, which can be an asset when the tape is used in areas particularly sensitive to alteration and impairment of circulation.

Great care must be taken in the preparation of the area to be taped in order to minimize the possibility of infection or irritation of the soft tissues involved. This precaution is particularly important if that area is the site of frequent reapplication of taping materials. Abrasions or cuts in the taping field must be properly dressed. Lubricated gauze or sponge pads should be applied in areas of potential friction, such as the Achilles and anterior tibialis tendons, where they course over the ankle joint. Wrinkled tape or tape ends that roll back with sock wear can become other mechanical sources of increased pressure and friction, especially on skin surfaces subjected to weight-bearing stress.

Improper tape application pressure can also cause skin irritation, particularly because tape must be applied with the limb placed in a nonweight-bearing position. For example, allowance for metatarsal expansion during weight bearing must be considered when taping the ankle joint.

Tape application in a continuous, circular fashion not only can cause skin irritation but also can have a profound deleterious effect on the neurovascular integrity of the soft tissues, especially if used in an edematous area. For this reason, adhesive strapping should be applied in strips, with each strip overlapping the previous one by one half its width. Wrinkling or tape "skirts," resulting from tape's not conforming to the contours of the area involved, also create areas of unwanted pressure.

Chemical or allergic causes of skin and soft tissue discomfort may result from the individual's reactivity to the adhesive base of the spray adherent (which is recommended for enhancing the duration and degree of the tape support) or from the adhesive backing of the tape itself. This reactivity is accentuated if the skin has been recently shaved. A pretaping underwrap and a base of hypoallergenic tape can provide a buffer to skin reaction but may also significantly compromise the adhesive properties and ultimate strength of the tape support.[20] The optimum way to enhance tape stability is to apply the tape directly to skin not recently shaved and to prepare the skin with a taping adherent.

The patient receiving this type of support should be well counseled as to when and how the taping should be removed. Under no circumstances should the tape remain in place longer than is necessary to achieve the desired outcomes. Tape cutters specifically designed to afford a cutting edge within a protective handle or bandage scissors used with a lubricated tip should be made available to the individual for timely removal. The removal instrument should be used on the least-involved portion of the injured area. Once incised, the tape should then be peeled downward in the direction of hair growth and in a line parallel to the skin contour. Attempts to remove tape strip by strip not only are time-consuming but also may subject the soft tissues to unnecessary and potentially damaging forces. Immediate inspection of the area is an important part of this routine to ensure optimal skin and soft tissue integrity.

FOOT AND LOWER LEG TAPING AND PADDING TECHNIQUES

Great Toe Taping Technique

Biomechanical Rationale

Turf toe injuries result from forced hyperextension and valgus stress to the metatarsophalangeal joint of the great toe. This injury commonly results from athletic endeavors in which a soft shoe is worn and the surface of play is unforgiving, as is the case with artificial turf. Sesamoiditis, metatarsalgia, bunion formation, and hallux rigidus can result secondary to long-term inflammation.[72]

For inflammation management and rehabilitation, adhesive strapping is used to restrict terminal dorsiflexion range of motion and to buffer the valgus forces imposed. These goals are accomplished with a combination of longitudinal strips to splint the joint and spicas to bias the limited magnitude of motion to the desired planes.

Technique

PREPARATION. The patient is placed in a nonweight-bearing position with the foot resting off the edge of the treatment table. The skin is properly prepared as presented in the general principles section. A small bandage may be placed over the toenail if tape will encroach on this area. The toe is placed in a neutral position as previously described. Two anchor strips of 1.5-inch adhesive tape are placed with minimum pressure around the midshaft of the metatarsals. Such circumferential strips must allow for expansion in a weight-bearing position. These strips should overlap each other by approximately one half their width (Fig. 7–1A).

TAPE APPLICATION. Splinting strips of 1-inch adhesive tape are applied from the metatarsal anchor to the interphalangeal joint of the great toe. These strips sequentially overlap each other and are fanned from the dorsal to the plantar surface of the joint (Fig. 7–1B). Two 1-inch adhesive strips are then sequentially applied to form a spica originating from the dorsal surface of the lateral metatarsals, continuing across the metatarsophalangeal joint

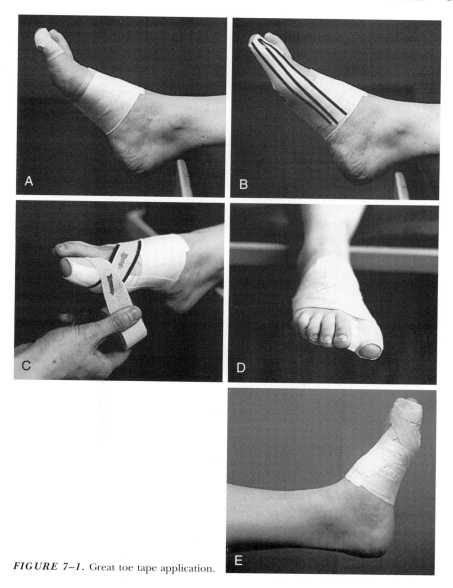

FIGURE 7–1. Great toe tape application.

(exerting pressure to limit extension), looping around the great toe, and then continuing across the plantar surface to terminate on the dorsum of the foot (Fig. 7–1C). In this manner the tape ends avoid the weight-bearing surface. The great and second toes may be taped together, or "buddy taped," with a felt piece placed between the toes to mechanically block the extremes of valgus stress on the joint (Fig. 7–1D). Adhesive 1.5-inch anchor strips seal the tape ends on the metatarsal region, finishing the procedure (Fig. 7–1E).

A stiffer shoe may be chosen for return to play. The shoe may be reinforced along the medial side of the inner toe box with a thermoplastic material. This material should be thin enough to minimize pressure within the confined space. Proper shoe fit accommodating the bulk of either the tape or the thermoplastic medial shoe liner is essential to the success of this treatment.

Low Dye Taping Techniques

Low dye taping is indicated in cases of medial arch strain, plantar fasciitis, metatarsalgia, and medial tibial stress syndrome (shin splints). Excessive or prolonged pronation combined with internal tibial rotation during weight bearing has been implicated as a biomechanical characteristic that may predispose the individual to the aforementioned conditions.[52] Heel and arch pain as well as inflammation of supinating musculature can result. Clement et al[18] attributed 75% of overuse running injuries to excessive pronation.

Biomechanical Rationale

The low dye techniques are theorized to directly control the foot and indirectly control the ankle and lower leg. This strapping procedure provides a more optimal posturing of the weight-bearing foot, thereby minimizing the development of these overuse injuries. The following techniques stabilize the metatarsal heads by holding them in a slight plantarflexed position, and they also support the medial longitudinal and transverse arches. The reverse figure-eight and medial heel-lock adjunctive techniques help to control extreme calcaneal valgus and internal tibial rotation believed to contribute to the mechanism of these overuse injuries.

Technique

PREPARATION. The patient is placed in a nonweight-bearing position with the foot extended off the table edge. The ankle is in zero degrees of dorsiflexion or in a neutral position. The foot is placed in a subtalar neutral position, and the toes are relaxed to a neutral position as well. The skin is prepared with an adherent taping base. Anchor strips are applied laterally to medially across the plantar aspect of the metatarsal heads. A 1-inch-wide moleskin strip is applied continuously from the distal anchor, laterally along the fifth metatarsal, around the posterior calcaneus at the Achilles tendon insertion, and then medially to the distal aspect of the first metatarsal.[85] Caution is used when the strips are placed across the calcaneus, and consistent placement at the tendinous insertion is emphasized. Placement of the strips distally onto the fat pad can result in low patient tolerance and resultant noncompliance (Fig. 7–2A).

TAPE APPLICATION. One-inch adhesive tape is applied to the plantar aspect of the fifth metatarsal. It extends over the moleskin anchor on the calcaneus, terminating medially on the plantar surface of the first metatarsal.

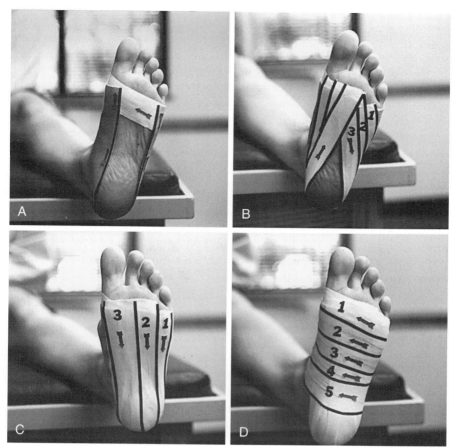

FIGURE 7–2. Low dye taping procedures.

Illustration continued on page 165

Subsequent strips overlapping the previous one are applied in a similar manner, fanning out from the fourth to the second metatarsal heads and from the third metatarsal head back to the same metatarsal head. Care is taken to apply proper tension in placing and sequentially molding the tape to the foot contour to ensure that the plantar soft tissues remain in a relative rest position. These fanned strips can vary in the origin and insertion sequence as case efficacy dictates[11] (Fig. 7–2B). Two to three overlapping longitudinal strips of 1.5-inch adhesive tape are then applied from the metatarsal heads to the calcaneal anchor, thereby supporting the medial longitudinal arch (Fig. 7–2C). Overlapping transverse strips of 1-inch adhesive tape are then applied laterally to medially beginning at the fifth metatarsal head and ending at the calcaneal tubercle, lending support to the transverse arch (Fig. 7–2D). The low dye procedure ends with a 1.5-inch adhesive tape anchor sealing the tape ends and mirroring the course of the moleskin. Two additional overlapping strips are then placed across the dorsum of the metatarsal region to further support the tape adherence (Fig. 7–2*E*). Weight-bearing testing of this taping is necessary to evaluate patient tolerance in a position of function.

Alternative taping materials can include the use of a moleskin strip cut out from a template drawn from the patient's foot dimensions. This moleskin strip is applied in lieu of adhesive tape but according to the same basic application principles (Fig. 7–2*F, G*). The moleskin approach is advocated if the additional bulk of the tape or the application of the low dye procedure proves to be a problem for the patient. These factors were frequently identified as limiting patients' compliance in home programs or regimens of self-care.[88]

Another alternative material highly regarded for its maintenance of adhesion over extended periods of wear is the rigid strapping tape and Hypafix (Smith & Nephew DonJoy, Inc., Carlsbad, CA).[56] This material has provided good results empirically when substituted for either the moleskin singular plantar strip or the 1-inch adhesive tape described in the original discussion of the low dye method.[65]

Medial Tibial Stress Syndrome Taping Techniques

Biomechanical Rationale

If further support beyond low dye taping is deemed necessary to control subtalar motion, as is usually the case in medial tibial stress syndrome, adjunctive procedures can be added to the low dye technique or can be used independently. These techniques can include the use of a 0.25-inch-thick and 1-inch-wide strip of felt placed along the distal third of the medial tibia to compress and minimize the theorized microtrauma to the tendinous insertional fibers along the periosteum[10] (Fig. 7–3*A*). To further support the medial soft tissue structures, both Grant[36] and Moss et al[58, 59] advocate stirrups applied with a lateral to medial tension intended to limit calcaneal eversion. Heel locks may also be applied to serve this purpose as well as to support the medial longitudinal arch. Moss and colleagues' approach is referred to as a reverse figure-eight.

Technique

PREPARATION. After tape adherent is applied to the affected skin, heel and lace pads with lubricant should be used over the anterior and posterior aspects of the ankle. These heel and lace pads conform to the joint contour and can be held in place with minimal application of underwrap. Two overlapping strips of 1.5-inch adhesive tape are applied as anchors just distal to the gastrocnemius muscle bellies (Fig. 7–3*B*).

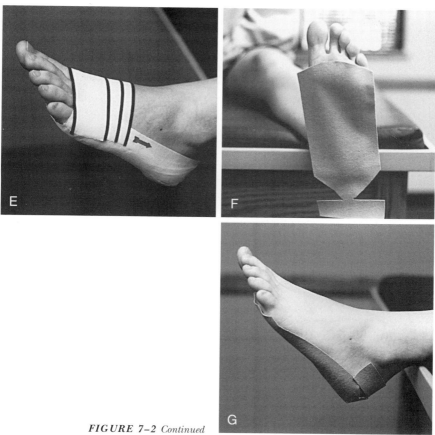

FIGURE 7–2 Continued

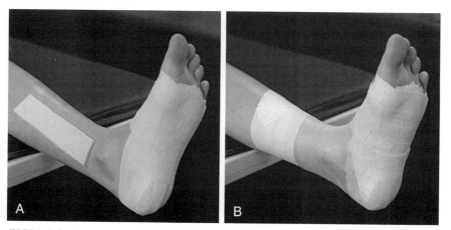

FIGURE 7–3. Medial tibial stress syndrome taping techniques.

Illustration continued on page 167

TAPE APPLICATION. Two stirrup strips running laterally to medially from anchor to anchor overlap and bisect the malleoli in their course. The reverse figure-eight strip can start laterally either on the anchor or at the lateral malleolus and can course under the arch, up across the instep, and over the dorsum of the ankle to overlap itself. It may end on the lateral malleolus to constitute one half of a figure-eight (Fig. 7–3C). Variations include continuing this strip to circumduct the malleoli posteriorly and then anteriorly emerging to cross the instep and to terminate along the medial tibia at the anchor. This method would constitute a full figure-eight (Fig. 7–3D). Either style of medial support is repeated with an overlapping piece. Subsequently a medial heel lock originating from the lateral malleolus courses across the medial malleolus and distal Achilles tendon. It then angles posteriorly to anteriorly across the lateral calcaneus with tension applied to limit calcaneal eversion. This strip terminates either across the instep to the medial anchor, consistent with a full figure-eight, or anteriorly across to its lateral malleolar origin (Fig. 7–3E). If the patient's history and clinical findings provide evidence of an inversion ankle sprain, a neutralizing lateral heel lock can be applied. This strip originates on the medial calcaneus, crosses the medial malleolus and anterior ankle toward the lateral malleolus, and circumducts the ankle posteriorly. Tension is applied at an anterior angle and is maintained across the plantar and medial calcaneus to prevent excessive calcaneal inversion. This strip terminates across the dorsum of the ankle at the medial calcaneal point of origin. Additional strips are applied from proximal to distal in a lateral to medial fashion, anchoring the preceding pieces and approximating the medial soft tissue structures (Fig. 7–3F, G). A weight-bearing evaluation of patient tolerance of this procedure should be performed, with adjustments made accordingly.

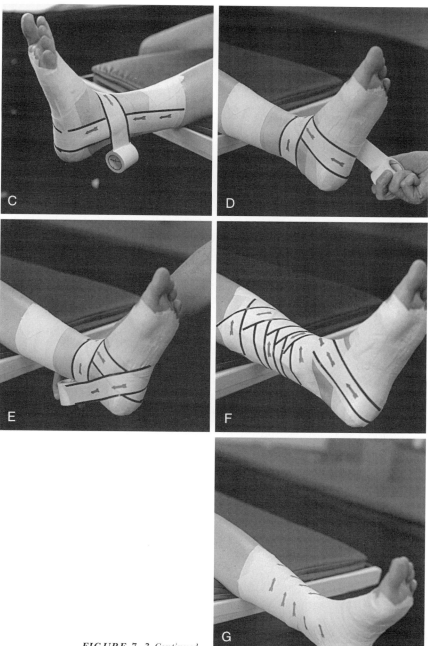

FIGURE 7–3 Continued

Effectiveness in Clinical Trials: Great Toe, Low Dye, and Medial Tibial Stress Syndrome Taping Techniques

The efficacy of the foot and lower leg taping and padding procedures has not been definitively established. Reproducible research is difficult to obtain owing to the variations in the type of tape used and in application technique.[26] Ferguson[24] questioned the efficacy of the use of adhesive tape and its duration of perceived effectiveness. Mobility of the skin as well as an increase in both perspiration produced by the tape and forces brought on by athletic activity destroy the integrity of this type of external support. Solutions to such problems have been offered by several studies. In 1993 Moss and associates[59] observed no significant decrease in support provided by either the low dye or the reverse figure-eight technique after subjects performed approximately 17 minutes of treadmill running. These authors attributed these results to improved taping preparation materials and procedures, as well as to the developmental advances in adhesive taping products and application techniques.

Specific to the application techniques presented, Scranton et al[75] used a force-plate analysis to study alterations in the support phase of walking when various means of external mechanical support were applied to the foot. Though low dye taping minimized the duration of forces under the midfoot, a rapid shift of these forces from the rearfoot to the forefoot was observed. This finding has obvious implications in individuals with metatarsalgia or a metatarsal stress fracture. Additionally, the authors reported that this means of support altered the weight-bearing forces to the extent that early symptoms of associated overuse syndromes were effectively managed.

DeLacerda,[21] Genuario,[32] and Brown et al[15] found a positive correlation between excessive pronation and the incidence of shin splints. All authors seemed to advocate some means of external support to modify the movement of the subtalar joint as a definitive treatment approach. Moss and associates[59] utilized two-dimensional film analysis to compare the effects of four different treatments on controlling the amount and the rate of foot pronation in athletes running on a treadmill. These treatments included low dye taping, reverse figure-eight stirrup taping, rigid orthoses, and no support. Rearfoot movement of calcaneal inversion or eversion relative to the lower leg in the frontal plane was quantified by digitization of high-speed film data. The authors found the reverse figure-eight taping to be the most effective taping technique to control the excursion of the calcaneus in the frontal plane.

Nawoczenski et al[61] advocated a three-dimensional analysis system to study movement patterns of the lower leg and rearfoot. Such techniques of analysis have yet to focus on the effect of the low dye and reverse figure-eight taping techniques on lower-leg and rearfoot kinematics during running.

Ankle Taping Techniques

The frequency with which ankle sprains are sustained is well documented in the literature. Barrett et al[7] reported that 10% to 28% of all sports-related injuries are ankle sprains. Rovere et al[70] stated that approximately 87% of ankle ligament sprains involve the lateral ligamentous complex. Garrick and Requa's[30] study concurred, identifying inversion ankle sprains as the most frequently occurring injury (estimated at 50%) in basketball. Ekstrand et al[23] reported that 17% of all soccer injuries were ankle sprains. Bosien et al[12] found that 33% of individuals who incurred ankle sprains demonstrated residual symptoms and peroneal weakness after injury. The finding was supported by Barrett et al,[7] who estimated that 20% to 50% of individuals with a history of ankle sprain exhibited some form of documented disability subsequently. Mack[53] offered a conservative estimate in reporting that 20% of those individuals with ankle sprains will develop chronic joint instability lasting 6 months or more after the initial injury.

General indications for use of adhesive strapping in ankle sprains can be categorized as *postinjury* to immobilize the extremity immediately, *prophylactic* to reduce the high incidence of reinjury, and *rehabilitative* to transcend the clinical course of injury management. This latter category is based on the theory that tape application enhances proprioceptive feedback, thereby increasing functional stability—a perception challenged in the literature subsequently reviewed.

Biomechanical Rationale

Abnormally severe or unexpected joint stresses may result in joint movement that exceeds normal physiologic limits, resulting in ligamentous sprains, capsular injury, and strain or subluxation of the peroneal tendons.[78] It is believed that tape application prevents joint movement beyond the physiologic limit of soft tissue strength. The exact amount of restriction of motion required to spare these structures is unknown or at least undocumented.

The goal of ankle taping is simply to provide an initial custom-fit orthosis designed to externally stabilize the subtalar joint, thereby protecting ligamentous and soft tissue structures without profoundly altering normal joint kinematics.[29] It is believed that the potentially injurious ankle inversion loads can be resisted by this enhanced mechanical stabilization. Injury is prevented by limiting the extremes of motion available, as well as by enhancing the neuromuscular response through the exteroceptive input provided by the tape.[8]

Technique

Ankle strapping or taping techniques are characterized by basic basket-weave, figure-eight, and heel-lock configurations designed to limit excessive tibiotalar and subtalar motion. Unless otherwise stated, these strapping techniques are presented as a means of preventing deleterious degrees of inversion stress to the lateral ankle ligaments. Adjunctive techniques and materials are numerous and are discussed after the standard technique description.

PREPARATION. The skin of the lower leg and ankle should be shaved and prepared with a tape adherent of known tolerance to the patient. Heel and lace pads with adequate lubricant can be applied to the Achilles tendon and the dorsum of the ankle. A protective underwrap can be applied circumferentially from the base of the fifth metatarsal to the lower one third of the leg where the gastrocnemius muscle bellies emerge. Anchors are placed circumferentially over the underwrap edges at the base of the muscle bellies and at the base of the fifth metatarsal (Fig. 7–4A).

TAPE APPLICATION. The standard taping method involves application of a basket weave using 1.5- to 2-inch porous tape woven in a sequence of overlapping strips. These strips alternate between a stirrup to support and limit frontal plane motion, a horseshoe strip to tether the stirrup distally, and an anchor strip to tether the stirrup proximally. These strips originate and terminate on the proximal anchor and are applied medially to laterally with the foot and ankle in a dorsiflexed and everted position (Fig. 7–4B).

After the basket weave has covered and has enclosed the ankle (Fig. 7–4C), an adjunctive technique, the subtalar sling, may be applied. This technique is described in a subsequent section.

The next part of the standard taping method requires the figure-eight stirrups to be applied. These strips begin medially, course over the anterolateral ankle, continue medially to the back of the ankle, laterally cross the dorsum of the foot, and finally terminate under the arch as a lateral stirrup (Fig. 7–4D, E). (Adjunctive procedures using various materials can be substituted at this point in the standard method. They are described in a subsequent section.) After two or three figure-eight bandages are applied, heel locks are added to further control subtalar motion. The lateral heel lock originates at a 45-degree angle laterally on the calcaneus (Fig. 7–4F). It

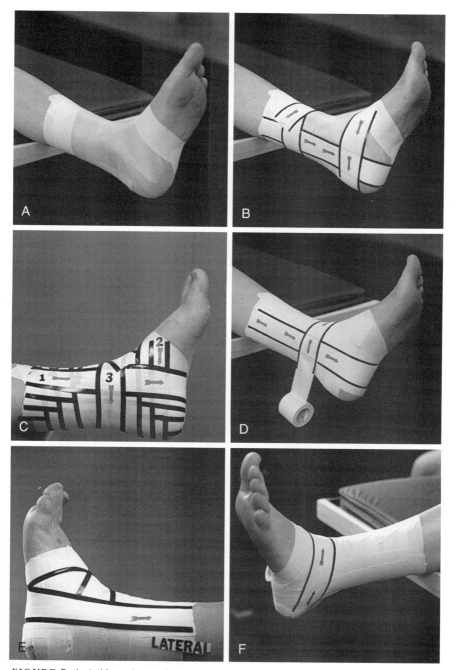

FIGURE 7–4. Ankle taping techniques.

Illustration continued on page 173

then courses across the front of the ankle, across and under the arch (Fig. 7–4*G*) to cross the lateral calcaneus (anchoring its origin there and pulling it into eversion), across the back of the ankle medially (Fig. 7–4*H*), and across the dorsum of the ankle to its lateral origin. The medial heel lock originates at a 45-degree angle at the medial calcaneus (Fig. 7–4*I*), courses anterolaterally across the lateral malleolus, and comes inferiorly across the medial calcaneus (anchoring its origin there), creating calcaneal eversion (Fig. 7–4*J*). The strip courses under the arch, up across the dorsum of the ankle, and back to terminate at its origin on the medial calcaneus. It is important to note here the bias of the calcaneus into eversion to assist in approximating the lateral ankle ligaments. However, these heel locks can truly "lock" the calcaneus in neutral if desired. The lateral heel lock is placed as described; the medial heel lock can be applied to course across the dorsum of the ankle toward the plantar aspect of the calcaneus, with tension applied across the medial calcaneus from inferiorly to superiorly. The strip then courses across the Achilles tendon over the anterior ankle to terminate where it originated (Fig. 7–4*K*).

The ankle taping is sealed proximally to distally with anchors to equalize pressure throughout and to optimize patient tolerance (Fig. 7–4*L*). Patient tolerance as well as the overall effectiveness of the tape is then assessed by having the patient bear weight on the ankle and attempt functional positions and movements.

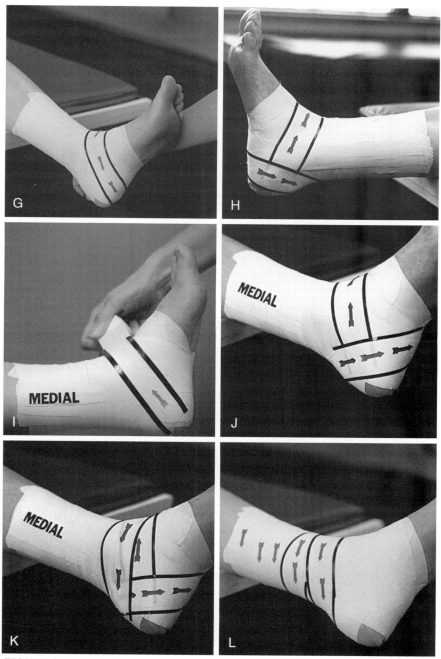

FIGURE 7–4 *Continued*

Illustration continued on page 175

ADJUNCTIVE TAPING TECHNIQUES. Various adjunctive techniques and materials can provide additional support for specific injury profile needs. These adjuncts include the use of DonJoy rigid strapping tape (Smith & Nephew DonJoy, Inc., Carlsbad, CA) to substitute for stirrup straps, because this material maintains good adhesion over an extended time.[56]

For greater rigidity in frontal plane restriction of movement, Hexcelite (Hexcel Medical Products, Dublin, CA) may be used for increased strength as well as for the convenience of remolding the stirrup as necessary. Its use may prove less costly than use of manufactured ankle stirrup orthoses.[47]

Moleskin may also serve as a substitute material to enhance the strength of stirrup support. Moleskin or 3-inch Elastikon (Johnson & Johnson, New Brunswick, NJ), with its elasticity reduced during application, may be applied as a stirrup from the proximal medial anchor, bisecting the medial malleolus and coursing under the calcaneus to the lateral malleolus (Fig. 7–4*M, N*). The tape could then be split down to this point, anchored over the anterolateral and posterolateral capsules respectively, and finally terminate around the proximal medial leg[41] (Fig. 7–4*O*). In this fashion, subluxing peroneal tendons can be tethered down and held posterior to the lateral malleolus.[74, 87] Other angles of split-stirrup anchoring may be attempted to achieve optimal stabilization results (Fig. 7–4*P*).

Another variation of stirrup application is offered by Moss et al.[58] Instead of the traditional origin of stirrup application on the medial proximal anchor, this approach originates on the anterolateral capsule. The strip then courses medially above the medial malleolus, across the back of the ankle, above the lateral malleolus, over the dorsum of the ankle, and under the arch to finally course laterally and to terminate as a traditional lateral stirrup.

For eversion ankle sprains, medial tibial stress syndrome, or shin splints, a reverse figure-eight is employed. This strip originates anteromedially, courses from above the lateral malleolus, courses around the ankle posteriorly, and continues across the dorsum of the ankle below the base of the fifth metatarsal, traveling under the arch to finally anchor on the medial proximal anchor of the leg.[59]

The subtalar sling described by Wilkerson[86] is a modified taping method that includes two strips of semielastic tape applied 45 degrees to the long axis of the foot in the sagittal plane. These overlapping strips originate on the plantar aspect of the metatarsal heads and course laterally and posteriorly to anchor around the posterior medial ankle (Fig. 7–4*Q*). This method adds more control of foot motion, providing greater limitation of inversion as compared with the standard taping technique. The greater control of inversion is achieved at a cost of greater restriction in plantarflexion, possibly resulting in a negative effect on performance. These strips may present a bowstring effect owing to the tension required in effective application. Dorsal forefoot anchoring strips may be required as part of the closure process to fasten these strips to the contour of the foot and ankle as well as to equalize pressure and to optimize patient tolerance.

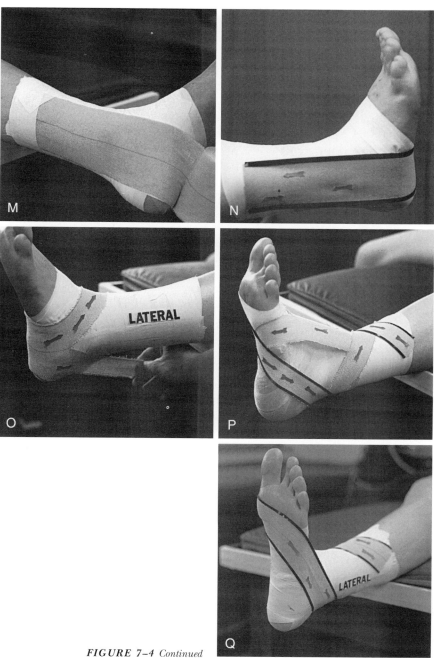

FIGURE 7–4 Continued

Effectiveness in Clinical Trials

More than any other technique of adhesive strapping and taping presented, those that involve supporting the ankle are the most frequently used and the most thoroughly studied to date. As a result, health care providers have greater objective data on which to base clinical decisions. However, many areas of controversy require substantiation by further clinical research.

Several studies have attempted to document the mechanical support provided by various taping materials and techniques of application and to quantify remaining residual support after imposition of exercise and functional activity. Overall, the level of tape support decreases with intensity and duration of activity. Possible explanations for inconsistencies reported in the literature may include variations in taping and testing, subject selection, and methodology of study.

Garrick and Requa[30] found benzoin skin preparation followed by application of zinc oxide tape directly to the skin to be the most effective for stability, although Andreasson et al[5] reported a 28% rate of skin problems with this method of tape application. Citing method of application as the determining factor in effectiveness of support, Garrick and Requa[30] found the tape/skin interface to be the weakest link in resistance to the mechanical stresses imposed. Pope et al[67] concurred with this finding in investigating which techniques provided the best mechanical support. It was determined that a force of 75 to 101 N is required for shear failure to occur at the tape/skin interface. Andreasson et al[4] reported that tape failure occurred at a force of 187 N; therefore, failure at the tape/skin interface would be expected to occur prior to actual tape failure. Pope et al[67] studied four different taping techniques applied to a wooden model of the tibiotalar and subtalar joints designed to articulate as torques were imparted to it at a controlled rate. A force of three times body weight applied at a distance of 0.2 meters to the laterally flexed ankle resulted in torques of 420 Nm. This finding was construed to be representative of dynamic loading incurred during athletic endeavors. Through use of a human model, the authors determined that angular displacement of the joints was tolerable to 7.6 degrees. The torque to failure was divided by this degree of tolerable angular displacement to arrive at measurable levels of angular stiffness. These levels provided sufficient resistance to applied loads while yielding a low angular displacement to stay within an athlete's tolerance. The necessary minimal level of stiffness, which was calculated to be 49.6 Nm, could be increased by adding additional layers of tape. The optimal stiffness configuration to withstand these loads was achieved by using the combination basket weave (horseshoe/basket weave/anchor technique) with three figure-eight straps. However, these authors acknowledged that the effects of repetitive cyclic loading on the yield stress of the various taping supports were not investigated. Bunch et al,[16] however, did demonstrate increased loss of taping support after 350 inversion cycles over a 20-minute period.

Mechanical stabilization afforded by taping techniques has been studied in terms of the range-of-motion restriction provided before athletic activity compared with that which remains after activity. Fumich et al[28] reported that the restrictive capacity of ankle taping dropped 40% after 10 minutes of exercise, but the remaining restriction endured 2 to 3 hours during subsequent physical activity. Whether this level of support was adequate to prevent injury was not determined. Myburgh et al[60] found that zinc oxide tape reduced the available range of motion up to 50% before exercise, but this support diminished to 30% restriction after 10 minutes of exercise and further weakened to only 10% restriction of motion after 1 hour of exercise. Elastic tape provided no inversion restriction after 10 minutes of exercise. Andreasson and Edberg[3] determined that ankle tape support was reduced 30% after 200 simulated running steps and 60% after 400 such steps. Greene and Hillman[37] reported that tape application restricted frontal plane movement by 41% of normal range, but this support lessened restriction of movement by 15% after 20 minutes of exercise.

Vaes et al[83] conducted a radiologic study of 51 athletes to assess the stabilization value of strapping the tibiotalar joint. Compared with elastic tape support involving figure-eight configuration, porous tape support of a basket weave, heel-lock, and figure-eight configuration demonstrated a statistically significant reduction in the talar tilt angle measured in a 40-degree plantarflexed position. This finding also held true after the subjects performed 30 minutes of agility activities. Lindley and Kernozek[50] reported residual range-of-motion restriction following a bout of exercise using the basket weave, moleskin stirrup, and heel-lock combination configuration. Rarick et al[68] determined that the basket weave, heel lock, and stirrup provided the best combination for support, although 40% of the initial restrictive quality was lost after 10 minutes of exercise. Wilkerson[86] advocated the addition of a subtalar sling to restrict frontal plane movement. The application of this adjunctive technique created greater control of foot motion compared with the standard technique. Residual range-of-motion restriction following exercise with the subtalar sling was 23% of normal plantarflexion values compared with 15% residual restriction with the standard taping technique alone. Additionally, residual restriction in supination and inversion ranges was 41% with the subtalar sling and 21% with the standard taping method. Wilkerson also reported that this same restriction pattern was observed after 2- to 3-hour football practices. Gross et al[38] found that this taping technique was at least equivocal to bracing in controlling passive frontal plane motion after exercise. Wilkerson's subtalar sling technique amounts to additional support to control inversion, but at a cost of slightly greater restriction of plantarflexion, which may have an impact on athletic performance capabilities. However, such a greater level of support may be indicated for recent injury or for the chronically unstable ankle.

Adhesive Strapping Versus Orthotic Intervention

Some researchers have investigated the effects of tape versus bracing in controlling ankle inversion. Gross et al[39] observed that ankle taping was similar to the Aircast Brace (Aircast, Inc., Summit, NJ) in the degree of inversion restriction remaining after exercise. Hughes and Stetts[43] reported ankle taping to be equivalent to semirigid braces in the retention of frontal plane support after exercise. Scheuffelen et al[73] imposed inversion moments to the ankle in positions of 20 to 30 degrees of plantarflexion to determine the efficacy of bracing versus taping invervention. Both brace and tape support were effective in reducing inversion motion, but neither method eliminated it. Rovere et al[71] advocated taping the ankle before application of an Aircast Brace to afford extra support during the early stages of injury.

Some clinicians have attempted to correlate shoe style and the perceived support afforded by tape with the incidence of ligamentous injury. Garrick[29] documented a low rate of ankle sprains in basketball players who were taped and who wore high-top sneakers. Barrett et al[7] concluded that there was no significant relationship between shoe type and ankle sprain. Ottaviani et al[62] examined the combined restraint provided by peroneal muscle activity and the wearing of high-top sneakers in controlling inversion motion at the ankle. Wearers of high-top sneakers showed an increase in inversion movement to 29.4% at 0 degrees of plantarflexion and 20.4% at 16 degrees of plantarflexion. In a cadaveric study in which the dynamic stabilizers were not included in the analysis of restraining forces, Shapiro et al[76] demonstrated that high-top sneakers improved the efficacy of tape support. Colville et al[19] noted the average electromyographic (EMG) peroneal muscle response time to a sudden inversion force to be 69 msec. Because of such neuromuscular latencies, the ankle may have to rely solely on passive restraints until dynamic stabilizers respond with sufficient force generation to prevent injury.

Effects on Functional Performance

The effect of ankle taping on functional performance has been well documented in the literature. Greene and Hillman[37] found that neither bracing nor ankle taping affected the vertical leap in volleyball players throughout 3 hours of play. Hamill et al[40] reported no negative effects on performance in base running with athletes whose ankles were supported by tape. However, Abdenour et al[1] and Gehlsen et al[31] reported a decrease in plantarflexion torque output, possibly attributed to a reduction in functional performance, in subjects with taped ankles. Burks et al[17] found that ankle taping significantly decreased athletic performance as manifested by a 4% decrement in vertical excursion, a 3.5% decrement in sprint time, and a 1.6% decrement in shuttle run time. MacKean et al[65] concurred with Burks et al[17] that vertical jump height was significantly impaired with use of ankle tape support. No decrements in motor tasks such as balance[48, 64] or agility[55, 63, 79, 84, 92, 97] have been reported under tape support conditions. Robinson et al[69] concluded that ankle tape support adversely affected agility test performance.

Proprioceptive Effects

One of the generally accepted tenets of ankle sprain rehabilitation is to improve the responsiveness and force production of the dynamic stabilizers of the ankle and foot. In the case of inversion stress, for example, the peroneal muscles become a focus of the rehabilitation program. The question arises as to the influence of tape support on the performance of this supportive musculature. Karlsson et al[46] suggested that tape works by shortening the peroneal reaction time through affecting proprioceptive function of ligaments and the joint capsule. Löfvenberg et al[51] documented EMG activity of peroneal muscles in 15 ankles characterized as chronically unstable and compared this activity with controls after imposition of sudden inversion stress. The symptomatic ankles demonstrated significantly longer ipsilateral reaction times (65 msec) than stable ankles (49 msec). Although the general belief holds that tape support stimulates skin receptors, which reflexively facilitate muscle contraction, the literature indicates that this theory may be difficult to prove definitively.

With the use of tape support, Scheuffelen et al[73] found that EMG readings of peroneal activation in response to controlled inversion moments were comparable to readings under physiologic conditions and were not correlated to the degree of inversion displacement. Sprigings and Pelton[78] compared tape-supported ankles with untaped ankles in EMG-monitored peroneal reaction to sudden weight-bearing inversion stress. No significant difference was noted. However, there was a tendency for the peroneal musculature to show the most activity without tape support and the least activity under tape support conditions. In three of four subjects, all of whom had a significant amount of talar tilt, Glick et al[34] found that the peroneus brevis function in the tape-supported subjects was prolonged at the end of the swing phase. This pattern served to position the foot in less inversion at initial contact. Interestingly, the degree of inversion at initial contact is thought to be excessive in most of those who incur inversion ankle sprains of the lateral ligaments.[25]

Karlsson and Andreasson's 1992 study[45] involved analysis of stress radiographic views of talar tilt and anterior talar translation of both stable and unstable ankles in 20 athletes. This radiographic analysis was performed with and without tape support. When results were compared, there was no significant reduction in the radiographic indicators of instability with or without tape support. In response to a simulated ankle inversion sprain mechanism, reaction time as measured by an EMG signal of the peroneal musculature was significantly slower in the unstable ankles of the 20 athletes than in the stable, contralateral limbs. The peroneal reaction time significantly improved with tape but did not equal that of the uninvolved ankles. Because athletes with the highest degrees of instability improved their reaction time the most significantly with tape support, the authors concluded that the tape must serve both to mechanically restrict ankle range of motion and to facilitate proprioceptive input. Although the authors believed that ankle tape support shortened the peroneal reaction time, a rationale was not offered for the observation that reaction time was not shortened in athletes with tape support who demonstrated low-grade mechanical instability.

Some authors have studied the effect of tape application on ankle proprioception and position sense. Although Dellon[22] suggested that position sense depends primarily on cutaneous sensibility, the literature questions the influence of tape support on exteroceptive information and proposed resultant behaviors such as postural control. Tropp et al[82] compared the postural equilibrium of 38 soccer players as assessed by stabilometry, a quantification of a modified Romberg test. When these subjects were tested with tape support, no significant impact on these scores was observed. The trend, however, was toward improvement of scores when tape support was applied.

By contrast, Thompson,[80] using a digital balance evaluator to assess dynamic balance and a modified Romberg test to assess static balance, observed that tape adversely affected postural control in 17 football players. Using a force platform, Bennell and Goldie[8] confirmed that tape support adversely affected the balance of 20 normal subjects when they were denied visual input. However, with visual input, these tape-supported subjects demonstrated no deficits. Bennell and Goldie theorized that in single-leg tape support, the normal kinematics of the foot and ankle necessary for proprioceptive input are insufficient to trigger the rapid responses to maintain postural control. Altered movement strategies are then substituted, and the skill needed to maintain normal responses theoretically deteriorates.

Goldie et al[35] documented postural control deficits of 8 weeks' duration in subjects who had sustained an inversion injury to the ankle. A similar group who practiced single-leg stance and specific balance exercises demonstrated no residual postural control deficits. Tropp et al[81] found that prophylactic ankle taping was no more effective than coordination training in postural control performance. Coordination training alone improved functional stability and postural control, resulting in a reduced incidence of ankle sprains. Freeman and Wyke[27] reported reduced rates of instability episodes after subjects performed a treatment program emphasizing coordination exercises.

Achilles Tendon Taping Techniques

Biomechanical Rationale

Adhesive strapping techniques involving the Achilles tendon are designed to restrict the functional length of the tendon, thereby reducing both the total amount of force potentially generated by the musculature and the resultant strain of the tendon. The ankle is placed in a slight plantarflexion position to achieve and to maintain this relative rest position. Achilles tendinitis and a partial tear of the tendon are two conditions for which these taping procedures could be included as part of the rehabilitation program.

Technique

PREPARATION. The skin is prepared with an adhesive taping base circumferentially applied to the proximal calf region and to the metatarsal region. Elastic tape of 2- to 3-inch width is utilized for the taping procedure.

A lubricated gauze pad is applied to the course of the Achilles tendon. Felt pads may be placed on each side of the tendon to decrease its potential for irritation from the taping procedure. The ankle is positioned in slight plantarflexion (Fig. 7–5A).

TAPE APPLICATION. Originating on the proximal anchor, a posteriorly centered strip of elastic tape courses distally, molding to the calcaneus and to the plantar aspect of the foot before terminating at the anchor on the metatarsal region. Two additional strips of elastic tape are applied in a similar fashion, but originating from the medial and lateral gastrocnemius heads to the lateral and medial aspects of the distal plantar anchor, respectively. After additional strips are applied to anchor the tape ends of these longitudinal strips, a securing bandage of 3-inch elastic tape may be

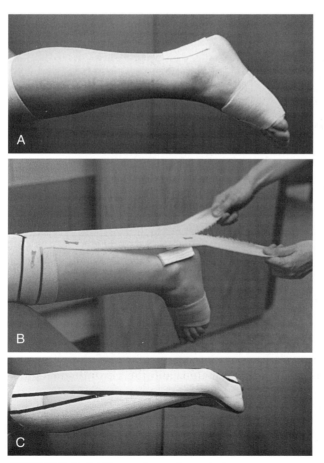

FIGURE 7–5. Achilles tendon taping technique.

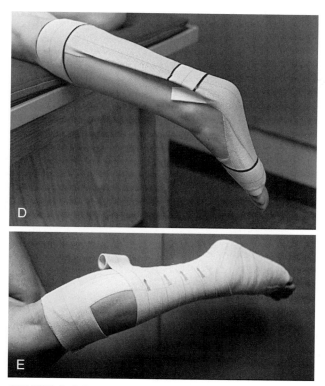

FIGURE 7–5 *Continued*

applied to isolate these strips from the subcutaneous tendon, thereby alleviating pressure and irritation. Alternatively, a circumferential wrap of 3-inch elastic tape may be placed distally to proximally, enclosing the entire tape support. The manner in which the relative elasticity is applied, however, must afford the individual the range of motion for the prescribed level of function. This tape application must be evaluated in a weight-bearing position with modifications made accordingly (Fig. 7–5*B* through *E*).

PATELLOFEMORAL TAPING TECHNIQUES

Health care practitioners have long attempted to reduce, if not eliminate, patellofemoral pain by repositioning the patella and thereby influencing the length-tension relationship of its periarticular tissues. Both bracing and taping techniques have been used individually or in combination to this end. Customized taping techniques constitute just one facet of McConnell's broader treatment program, which incorporates alteration of faulty lower-extremity biomechanical characteristics as well as achievement of optimal patellar orientation.[56] Normalization of patellar orientation allows retraining of dynamic patellar stabilizers in order to maintain a response of proper timing and force production to meet imposed weight-bearing demands. Although McConnell reported a 96% rate of effectiveness in ameliorating patellofemoral pain, reliability studies concerning the specific taping techniques employed as part of the program are few. Gerrard[33] conducted a clinical trial utilizing the McConnell program and reported that 86% of individuals with patellofemoral pain resumed and retained pain-free normal activity at a 12-month follow-up point. No control group was used, and objective data to substantiate such results were not offered.

Biomechanical Rationale

Characteristics of patellar position include glide, tilt, and rotation. As abnormal patellar postures are assessed, tape is applied to reorient the patella to approximate a more normal alignment. Subsequent functional training and testing results assist in refining the tension and angulation needed to allow pain-free function.

Technique

PREPARATION. Tape adherent is applied to the previously shaved skin. Hypafix is applied with minimal tension from medial to lateral over the patellofemoral joint (Fig. 7–6A).

TAPE APPLICATION. Rigid strapping tape is then applied to bias the patella in such a manner as to correct the malalignment features previously assessed. Lateral patellofemoral compression syndrome may be treated with a medially biased strip that shifts the patella medially in the frontal plane and medially along the longitudinal axis (Fig. 7–6B). This approach attempts to decompress the lateral tilt patellar posture and to distract the abnormally shortened lateral retinacular tissues that characterize this syndrome. Patellar internal or external rotation may be corrected with strips that are applied to derotate the inferior or superior pole (Fig. 7–6C, D). Patellar baja may be treated by decompressing the inferior pole and by reducing its pressure onto the infrapatellar fat pad (Fig. 7–6E). A tape strip that decompresses the superior pole and that assists in superior migration of the patella may be placed over a tape roll used as a fulcrum to assist this effort (Fig. 7–6F). This approach is often needed in a program to correct extension contracture of the knee.

Inherent in these attempts to improve patellar position is assessment of dynamic control of this joint. Open versus closed kinetic chain assessment should be part of this individualized evaluation of taping efficacy. Functional movement includes components of both weight-bearing and nonweight-bearing phases and positions.

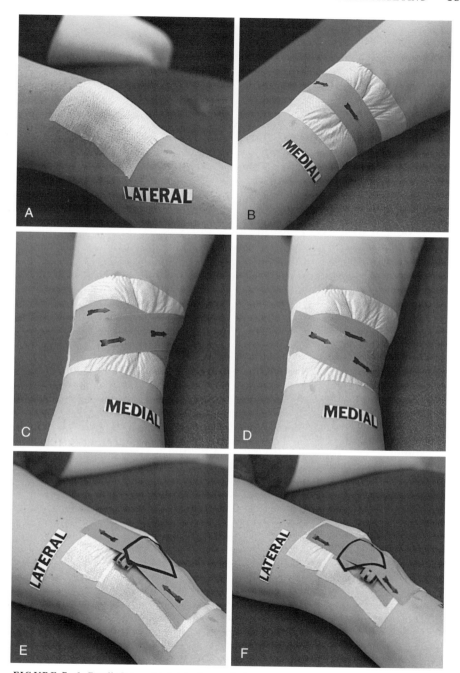

FIGURE 7–6. Patellofemoral joint taping techniques.

Effectiveness in Clinical Trials

As with previous taping techniques presented, the variables of application angle and tensioning, tape adherence quality and duration, tape tensile strength, and methodology of overall treatment approach may discourage quantification in research investigations regarding the efficacy of this procedure. However, Brockrath et al[14] attempted to document and to quantify the impact of patellar taping in terms of change in the patellofemoral congruence angle. Although no significant change in patellar alignment was observed, patellar taping decreased pain by approximately 50%. Larsen et al[49] examined the patellofemoral congruence angle in 20 asymptomatic men to evaluate the effect of the medial taping technique before and after exercise. Radiographic documentation of patellar position was studied at 40 degrees of knee flexion in a weight-bearing position. The baseline patellofemoral congruence angle of the untaped knee following exercise indicated a significant lateral shift of 4.6 degrees beyond midline. The average medial patellar shift after taping was 9 degrees medially beyond midline. After exercise, this medial shift was 0.57 degrees. Although this finding may indicate a substantial failure of the tape support, the maintenance of medial bias actually indicated some degree of efficacy of this technique.

PATELLAR TENDON TAPING AND PADDING TECHNIQUES

Overuse syndromes such as patellar tendinitis may result from a myriad of biomechanical factors that, combined with improper training techniques involving repetitive quadriceps contraction, will be manifest as signs and symptoms of inflammation. The tendon is commonly involved either at the inferior pole of the patella or at the insertion of the tendon at the tibial tubercle. During adolescence, with its periods of rapid growth, stress transmitted through the extensor mechanism may cause repeated microtrauma to the growth center. Apophysitis at the tibial tubercle may result and could lead to secondary heterotopic bone formation, commonly referred to as Osgood-Schlatter disease.

Biomechanical Rationale

Either taping or protective padding techniques may be employed to protect this portion of the extensor mechanism. A counterforce band may limit some of the force transmission and may place the inflamed area in a relative rest position. The same rationale is generally accepted in the use of a protective Plastazote (Apex Foot Products, South Hackensack, NJ) or horseshoe pad custom-made for protection of the tibial tubercle.

Techniques

PREPARATION. The infrapatellar area should be shaved and a tape adherent applied. The knee is placed in a position of slight flexion. A minimally lubricated gauze pad may be placed across the posterior capsule. Underwrap use is optional.

TAPE APPLICATION. A 1-inch strip of elastic tape is applied with gentle pressure circumferentially around the knee, capturing the optional protective posterior capsule pad and the patellar tendon. Two or three additional strips may be used, with each directly overlapping the prior strip so as not to contact either the distal pole of the patella or the tibial tubercle. Weight-bearing repetitive flexion and extension of the knee allows the patient to evaluate the placement and applied tension relative to effectiveness and comfort level. Proper distal neurovascular status must be part of the taping technique tolerance evaluation (Fig. 7–7).

PAD FABRICATION. A circular Plastazote pad is cut to the dimensions to encircle the tibial tubercle, and the inner tubercle dimension is cored. This donut pad is placed in a convection oven at 300 to 350°F. With the affected area wrapped lightly by a protective elastic wrap, the patient is placed in a weight-bearing position of 30 degrees of knee flexion, and the heat-moldable pad is placed over the wrap-protected area. Elastic wrap is then used to help form the pad to the contour of the area. The pad is allowed to cool and to harden in a functional position. The inner core initially removed is then used to provide a relief area in the outer pad. A layer of heat-softened thermoplastic material is placed over the inner core protrusion and is secured with the elastic wrap until the outermost layer cools and hardens. The inner core is then removed, and the pad is trimmed. The thermoplastic

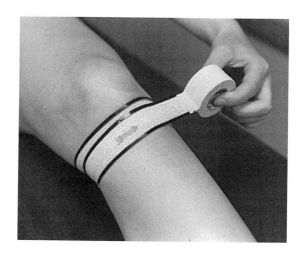

FIGURE 7–7. Patellar tendon taping technique.

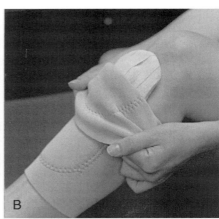

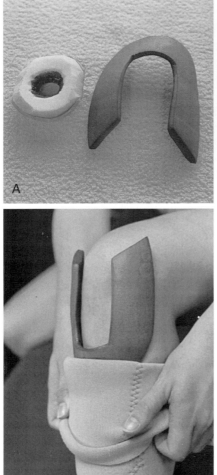

FIGURE 7–8. Patellar tendon pad fabrication.

shell can be joined to its softer inner Plastazote pad with tape (see Fig. 7–11*A* through *D*).

PAD APPLICATION. The pad is then placed over the tibial tubercle and is held by a nylon or neoprene sleeve. This pad affords not only a relief area of the inflamed apophysis but a counterforce compression over the patellar tendon with its moderation of extensor force transmission.

As an alternative approach, a horseshoe-shaped Plastazote pad may be molded in a manner similar to that of the circular pad. It is placed over the area as an upright U positioned around the tibial tubercle. The uprights of this horseshoe assist in patellar alignment and tracking. It too can be held in place with a supportive sleeve. It does not, however, offer the hardened thermoplastic shell, which may prove advantageous in the prevention of contusion of the area (Fig. 7–8).

KNEE TAPING TECHNIQUES

The following taping techniques have been devised to provide customized support to the knee joint. These adhesive strapping applications can be used either alone or in combination with knee braces in an effort to maximize static stabilization of the joint complex as well as to elicit a more responsive dynamic stabilization response to protect this area.

Posterior Capsule Support Technique

Biomechanical Rationale

The purpose of this taping technique is to prevent hyperextension (end-range extension) of the knee, thereby protecting the posterior capsule and related structures from injury or exacerbation of existing injury. This technique can be considered an adjunctive technique to anterior cruciate ligament protection.

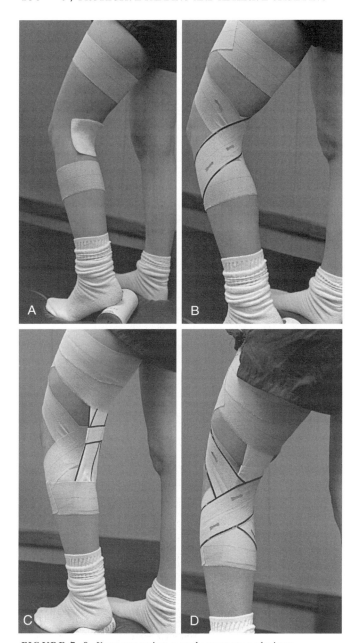

FIGURE 7-9. Knee posterior capsule support technique.

Technique

PREPARATION. A gauze with lubricant is applied to the popliteal fossa of the previously shaved knee. Anchor strips of 3-inch elastic tape are lightly applied circumferentially to the proximal thigh and the mid lower leg. If the anchors are placed at greater distances from the popliteal fossa, improved leverage can be gained through the supporting tape strips. Underwrap application is optional. The knee is positioned in 30 to 40 degrees of flexion (Fig. 7–9A).

TAPE APPLICATION. Three-inch elastic tape is applied in a spiral from the anteromedial tibial anchor across the posterior capsule, terminating anterolaterally on the proximal anchor. A second spiral strip is applied from the anterolateral tibial anchor to mirror the course of the first spiral, ending anteromedially on the proximal anchor. Two additional anchors can then be applied proximally and distally to tether these spiral strips (Fig. 7–9B). A fan-shaped checkrein can be fashioned from 1.5- to 2-inch porous tape and can be applied with tension to maintain joint flexion (Fig. 7–9C). Two additional but optional spirals can then be applied as initially described (Fig. 7–9D). The patellar region can be left tape-free (Fig. 7–9E). Weight-bearing functional movements are used to assess strapping effectiveness and patient tolerance of this procedure.

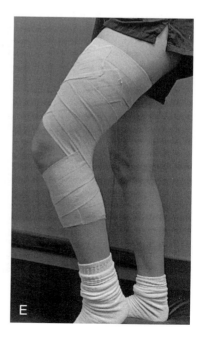

FIGURE 7–9 Continued

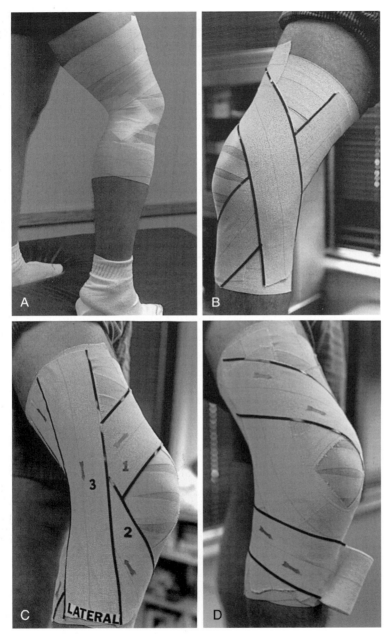

FIGURE 7–10. Collateral and anterior cruciate ligament tape support techniques.

Collateral and Anterior Cruciate Ligament Support Techniques

Biomechanical Rationale

The goal of collateral ligament taping procedures is to provide support to the medial and lateral ligaments in order to control valgus and varus angulation forces, respectively. Strips designated for anterior cruciate ligament protection are applied to limit anterior translation of the tibia.

Technique

PREPARATION. The knee is prepared in the same manner as in the prior technique (Fig. 7–10A).

TAPE APPLICATION. Three-inch elastic tape strips are initiated from the posteromedial distal anchor coursing parallel to the medial collateral ligament. Each strip crosses the tibiofemoral joint line and then courses along the anteromedial superior border of the patella. Each strip terminates anterolaterally on the proximal anchor. A strip of similar length originates on the anterolateral distal anchor, crosses the anteromedial inferior border of the patella, and parallels the medial collateral ligament. It terminates on the posteromedial proximal anchor (Fig. 7–10B). Two subsequent strips are applied in a similar manner for lateral collateral support. These strips are anchored again proximally and distally. Each medial and lateral X strip now formed is repeated for increased support and is placed to overlap its predecessor by two thirds its width (Fig. 7–10C). These strips are again anchored. Spiral strips may be placed from the proximal anteromedial anchor, coursing laterally to cross behind the posterior capsule, to emerge bisecting the anterior tibiofemoral joint line. They are then directed back

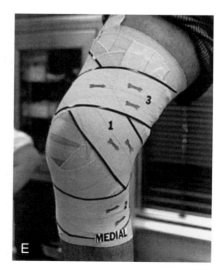

FIGURE 7–10 Continued
Illustration continued on following page

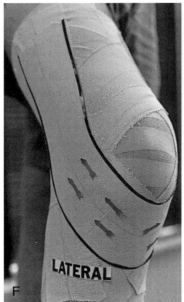

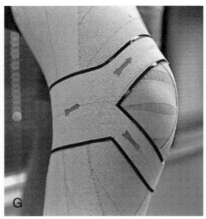

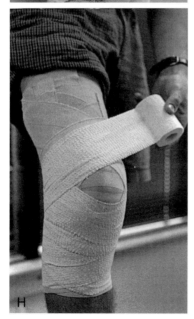

FIGURE 7–10 Continued

across the posterior capsule to terminate across the anteromedial thigh at the anterolateral anchor. A second figure-eight strip can be applied in the opposite (mirror) fashion to negate any bias of tibial rotation (Fig. 7–10*D*, *E*). A U-shaped piece of 3- to 4-inch elastic tape can then be applied across the anterior tibial plateau and subsequently anchored proximally (Fig. 7–10*F*). This is an adjunctive technique to minimize anterior tibial translation. A V-shaped piece of 3- to 4-inch elastic tape can also be applied across the posterior capsule and can be split to align the patella both medially and laterally (Fig. 7–10*G*). The technique is completed with lightly compressive wrap applied to equalize the pressure throughout the region and to secure the tape ends (Fig. 7–10*H*). Weight-bearing functional movements are then used to assess tape effectiveness and patient tolerance of this procedure.

Effectiveness in Clinical Trials

To date, published reports discussing the efficacy of knee taping techniques are relatively few. Anderson et al[2] reported that little is known about the impact of tape support in knee joint kinematics or its effectiveness as a static stabilizer in either injured or uninjured knees. Hunter[44] stated that there is no evidence to support the belief that taping techniques using a crisscross pattern of support actually provide an increase in joint stability. Although knee taping procedures provide a good custom fit, Morehouse[57] reported that any intended increase in medial capsular support rendered by the procedures had dissipated after just 5 minutes of intense exercise. Anderson et al's[2] cadaveric study compared two knee braces with tape support. The greatest reduction in anteroposterior displacement and internal/external rotation was provided by the combination of tape support under a Lenox Hill Brace (3M, Inc., Minneapolis, MN).

To what magnitude dynamic restraints provide protection and to what extent proprioceptive input plays a role in the stability of the knee have been the focus of related studies. Branch et al[13] found that even with brace support, the muscle firing patterns of the quadriceps, hamstrings, and gastrocnemius muscle groups in the anterior cruciate ligament–deficient knee did not change. Harman and Frykman[42] hypothesized that the perceived effectiveness of knee wraps was due to thermal effects and to an associated increase in blood flow as well as to enhancement of soft tissue pliability. Improved patellar alignment was also credited for elimination of pain-driven neural inhibition, thereby allowing greater muscle recruitment and force production. Through perception of the threshold of joint motion and reproduction of set joint angles, Perlau et al[66] studied inherent knee proprioception in 54 normal subjects. The authors reassessed proprioception immediately after an elastic bandage was applied, 1 hour later, and finally after its removal. Although the bandage wear improved proprioception during its use, the authors found no carryover after its removal. The proprioceptive impact of knee taping applications, if any, remains to be definitively determined.

LOWER AND UPPER LEG PADDING TECHNIQUES

Biomechanical Rationale

Padding for the leg is most commonly used for protection of contusions to the anterior compartment, after a hematoma is surgically decompressed through fascial release, or during a period of callus remodeling in healed lower-leg fractures. In the thigh region, the most frequent indication is protection of a quadriceps contusion to minimize the development of myositis ossificans or to protect a contused anterior superior iliac spine or iliac crest from direct contact. This approach to protection can transcend the phases of rest/rehabilitation and protected return to function.

Technique

PREPARATION. The area requiring protection is identified, and a Plastazote pad is cut to the appropriate circumference. The inner core is hollowed out, and the outer donut pad is placed in a 300° to 350°F convection oven to allow it to become moldable (Fig. 7–11A). The inner core is placed over the recessed relief area, and a heat-softened thermoplastic ⅛- to ¼-inch covering is applied over the protruding center pad and its circular base (Fig. 7–11B). The affected area is protected with an elastic wrap with enough length held in reserve to secure the warm pad to the anatomic contour of the leg (Fig. 7–11C). Once cooled, the inner core is removed, and the hardened thermoplastic shell is secured to its softer donut pad with tape (Fig. 7–11D). (As an adjunctive technique, bubble packing can be used under the thermoplastic shell.[77])

PAD APPLICATION. The means by which the pad is secured is area-dependent. The goal is to avoid pad migration, which can increase pressure on the contused area. Tape may assist in securing the pad to the lower leg. The emphasis is to minimize circumferential wrapping, which has an associated increased risk of elevated compartment pressure. The upper leg seems to tolerate circumferential elastic tape use in securing the protective pad (Fig. 7–11E). Alternatively, a heavy-grade spandex thigh girdle or sleeve can suffice for this purpose. Under no circumstances can distal neurovascular status be compromised.

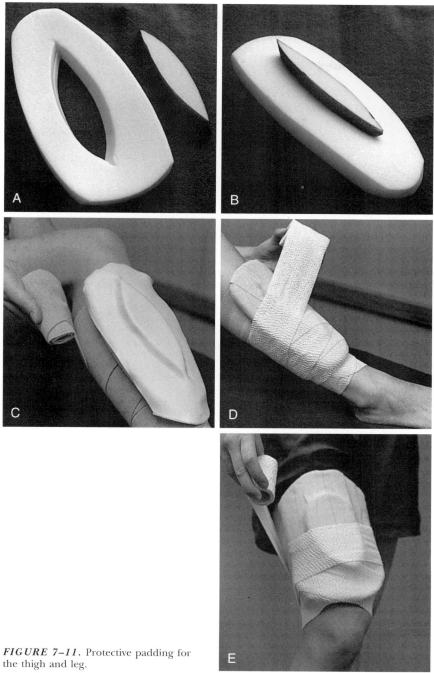

FIGURE 7–11. Protective padding for the thigh and leg.

THIGH AND HIP TAPING AND WRAPPING TECHNIQUES

Biomechanical Rationale

Tape and compression wrap support for the thigh and hip are indicated for soft tissue strains. The goal is to add compression support and to place the strained tissues in a relative rest position. These techniques minimize positions of passive insufficiency of the soft tissues during the rest/rehabilitative phase of recovery and the protected return to athletic activity.

Technique

PREPARATION. The area may be previously shaved and a tape adherent applied. Underwrap use is optional. A 6-inch-wide elastic wrap, usually of double length, is used. Pieces of porous tape may tag the starting end of the elastic wrap and may secure it to the leg. The wrap is held with the top layer most closely applied to the skin. In this manner, optimal control of tension application is realized.

WRAP APPLICATION. In all cases, the wrap is applied in a crisscross or V manner to minimize circumferential pressure and the heightened risk of neurovascular compromise. The patient is placed in a position of hip flexion, adduction, or extension (as dictated by the muscle groups involved), and a shortened or relative rest position is achieved.

For quadriceps or hip flexor strains, the patient is positioned in hip flexion, slight internal rotation, and midline alignment parallel with the sagittal plane. The wrap, which should be 6 inches wide and of double length (10 feet long), is anchored anterolaterally on the proximal thigh. It continues distally and medially, surrounding the leg posterolaterally, and then courses superior medially to anchor at its origin (Fig. 7–12A).

Tension is applied when wrapping posteriorly to anteriorly and when wrapping laterally to medially to bias the hip into flexion and toward the midline into slight adduction (Fig. 7–12B). This crisscross angulated application is repeated, each strip overlapping its preceding layer by about one half the width and moving proximally. Upon reaching the hip level, the wrap emerges posteriorly to anteromedially and is tightened and brought superiorly across the opposite iliac crest. The waist is then crossed posteriorly to arrive across the ipsilateral iliac crest and finally to cross in front of the anterior superior iliac spine. The wrap is then angulated distally to enclose the proximal thigh, and a second hip spica may be applied (Fig. 7–12C). The wrap end is secured with 2- to 3-inch-wide elastic tape that also repeats the hip spica pattern (Fig. 7–12D). This pattern of wrapping can also be used to secure protective pads fabricated for the anterior superior iliac spine or iliac crest contusions (Fig. 7–12E, F).

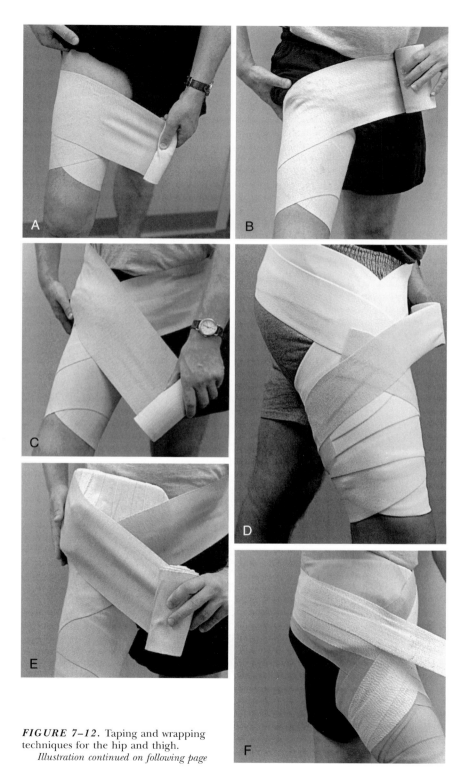

FIGURE 7-12. Taping and wrapping techniques for the hip and thigh.

Illustration continued on following page

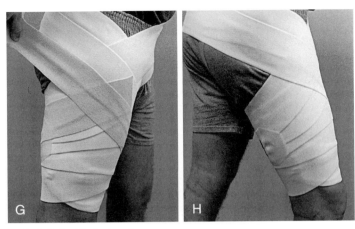

FIGURE 7–12 *Continued*

Hip adductor strains are supported in a similar manner, but with greater tension applied laterally to medially to approximate the adductor musculature. The position of the hip in the sagittal plane is dictated by which adductors are strained.

Hip extensor strains involving the proximal hamstrings or gluteus maximus muscle can also be placed in a protected position with an elastic hip spica wrapping. Application of selective tensioning places the bias of position and movement of the hip into extension (Fig. 7–12*G*).

An alternative material for use in these wrapping techniques is SuperWrap (Fabrifoam Products, Inc., Exton, PA). This material provides compression application capacity comparable to that of traditional elastic cloth wraps but reportedly resists migration because of a superior coefficient of friction (Fig. 7–12*H*).

SUMMARY

The taping techniques and protective padding fabrications presented in this chapter may be labor intensive in the initial trials of fabrication and application. However, with experience and skill development, these techniques give the practitioner invaluable tools with which to protect the individual from potentially deleterious stress.

REFERENCES

1. Abdenour TE, Saville WA, White RC, et al: The effect of ankle taping upon torque and range of motion. Athletic Training 15:227–228, 1979.
2. Anderson K, Wojtys EM, Loubert PV, et al: A biomechanical evaluation of taping and

bracing in reducing knee joint translation and rotation. Am J Sports Med 20(4):416–421, 1992.

3. Andreasson G, Edberg B: Rheological properties of medical tape used to prevent athletic injuries. Textile Res J 53(4):225, 1983.
4. Andreasson G, Edberg B, Peterson L, et al: Mechanical functional analysis of tape. Lakartidningen 77(41):3628, 1980.
5. Andreasson G, Reese D, Renstrom P: Subjective experience of medical tape used to prevent athletic ankle injuries. Thesis. Department of Textile Technology, Chalmers University of Technology, Göteborg, Sweden, 1985.
6. Arnheim, DD: Modern Principles of Athletic Training, 7th ed, Philadelphia, W.B. Saunders Co., 1989.
7. Barrett JR, Tanji JL, Drake C, et al: High vs. low-top shoes for the prevention of ankle sprains in basketball players. A prospective randomized study. Am J Sports Med 21(4):582–585, 1993.
8. Bennell KL, Goldie PA: The differential effects of external ankle support on postural control. J Orthop Sports Phys Ther 20(6):287–295, 1994.
9. Birrer RB, Poole B: Taping of sports injuries: Review of a basic skill. J Musculoskel Med 11(6):56–68, 1994.
10. Bisek AM: Shin splint taping: Something extra. Athletic Training 22(3):216, 1987.
11. Bissonnette KA, Leard JS: Variation of the longitudinal arch strapping. Athletic Training 17(1):30, 1982.
12. Bosien WR, Staples AS, Russel SW: Residual disability following acute ankle sprain. J Bone Joint Surg 37A:1237–1243, 1955.
13. Branch TP, Hunter R, Donath M: Dynamic EMG analysis of anterior cruciate deficient legs with and without bracing during cutting. Am J Sports Med 17(1):35–41, 1989.
14. Brockrath K, Wooden C, Worrell T, et al: Effects of patella taping on patella position and perceived pain. Med Sci Sports Exerc 25:989–992, 1993.
15. Brown TD, Van Hoeck JE, Brand RA: Laboratory evaluation of prophylactic knee brace performance under dynamic valgus loading using a surrogate leg model. Clin Sports Med 9:751–762, 1990.
16. Bunch RP, Bednarski K, Holland D, et al: Ankle joint support: A comparison of reusable lace-on braces with taping and wrapping. Physician Sportsmed 13(5):59–62, 1985.
17. Burks RT, Bean BG, Marcus R, et al: Analysis of athletic performance with prophylactic ankle devices. Am J Sports Med 9(2):104–106, 1991.
18. Clement DB, Taunton JE, Smart GW, et al: A survey of overuse running injuries. Physician Sportsmed 9(5):47–58, 1981.
19. Colville MR, Marder RA, Boyle JJ, et al: Strain measurement in lateral ankle ligaments. Am J Sports Med 18:196–200, 1990.
20. DeLacerda F: Effect of underwrap conditions on the supportive effectiveness of ankle strapping with tape. J Sports Med Phys Fitness 18:77–81, 1978.
21. DeLacerda F: A study of anatomical factors involved in shinsplints. J Orthop Sports Phys Ther 2(2):125–131, 1980.
22. Dellon AL, Curtis RM, Edgerton MT: Re-education of sensation in the hand after nerve injury and repair. Plast Reconstr Surg 53:297, 1974.
23. Ekstrand J, Gillquist J, Liljedahl S: Prevention of soccer injuries. Am J Sports Med 11:116–120, 1983.
24. Ferguson AB: The case against taping. J Sports Med 1:46–47, 1973.
25. Firer P: Effectiveness of taping for prevention of ankle ligament sprains. Br J Sports Med 24(1):47–50, 1990.
26. Frankeny JR, Jewett DG, Hanks GA, et al: A comparison of ankle-taping methods. Clin Sports Med 3:20–25, 1993.
27. Freeman MAR, Wyke B: Articular reflexes at the ankle joint: An electromyographic study of normal and abnormal influences of ankle-joint mechanoreceptors upon reflex activity in the leg muscles. Br J Surg 54:990–1001, 1967.
28. Fumich RM, Ellison AE, Guerin GJ, et al: The measured effect of taping on combined foot and ankle motion before and after exercise. Am J Sports Med 9:165–170, 1981.
29. Garrick JG: The frequency of injury, mechanism of injury and epidemiology of ankle sprains. Am J Sports Med 5:241, 1977.
30. Garrick JG, Requa RK: Role of external support in the prevention of ankle sprains. Med Sci Sports Exerc 5:200–203, 1973.

31. Gehlsen GM, Pearson D, Bahamonde R: Ankle joint strength, total work, and range of motion: Comparison between prophylactic devices. Athletic Training 26:62–65, 1991.
32. Genuario SE: Differential diagnosis: Exertional compartment syndromes, stress fractures, and shin splints. Athletic Training 24(1):31–33, 1989.
33. Gerrard B: The patellofemoral pain syndrome: A clinical trial of the McConnell programme. Aust J Physiother 35:71–80, 1989.
34. Glick JM, Gordon RB, Nishimoto D: The prevention and treatment of ankle injuries. Am J Sports Med 4:136–141, 1976.
35. Goldie PA, Evans OM, Bach TM: Postural control following inversion injuries of the ankle. Phys Med Rehabil 75:969–975, 1994.
36. Grant JD: Taping for medial tibial stress syndrome. Athletic Training 25(1):53–54, 1990.
37. Greene TA, Hillman SK: Comparison of support provided by a semirigid orthosis and adhesive taping before, during, and after exercise. Am J Sports Med 18(5):498–506, 1990.
38. Gross MT, Batten AM, Lamm AL, et al: Comparison of DonJoy Ankle Ligament Protector and subtalar sling ankle taping before and after exercise. J Orthop Sports Phys Ther 19(1):33–41, 1994.
39. Gross MT, Lapp AK, Davis JM: Comparison of Swede-O-Universal ankle support and Aircast Sport Stirrup orthoses and ankle tape in restricting ankle eversion-inversion before and after exercise. J Orthop Sports Phys Ther 13(1):11–19, 1991.
40. Hamill J, Knutzen KM, Bates BT, Kirkpatrick G: Evaluation of two ankle appliances using ground reaction force data. J Orthop Sports Phys Ther 1986, 7:204–249.
41. Harbottle J: A comparison of adhesive ankle strappings. Athletic Training 19(1):72–73, 1983.
42. Harman E, Frykman P: The effects of knee wraps on weightlifting performance and injury. JNSCA 12(5):30–35, 1990.
43. Hughes LH, Stetts DM: A comparison of ankle taping and a semi-rigid support. Physician Sportsmed 11(4):99–103, 1983.
44. Hunter GY: Braces and taping. Clin Sports Med 4(3):439–454, 1985.
45. Karlsson J, Andreasson GO: The effect of external ankle support in chronic lateral ankle joint instability: An electromyographic study. Am J Sports Med 20(3):257–261, 1992.
46. Karlsson J, Sward L, Andreasson GO: The effect of taping on ankle stability: Practical implications. Sports Med 16(3):210–215, 1993.
47. Knue J, Hitchings E: The use of rigid stirrup for prophylactic ankle support. Athletic Training 22(2):121, 1982.
48. Kozar W: Effects of ankle taping upon dynamic balance. Athletic Training JNATA 9:11–13, 1974.
49. Larsen R, Andreasen E, Urfer A, et al: Patellar taping: A radiographic examination of the medical glide technique. Am J Sports Med 23(4):465–471, 1995.
50. Lindley TR, Kernozek TW: Taping and semirigid bracing may not affect ankle functional range of motion. JNATA 30(2):109–112, 1995.
51. Löfvenberg R, Karrholm J, Sundelin G, et al: Prolonged reaction time in patients with chronic lateral instability of the ankle. Am J Sports Med 23(4):414–417, 1995.
52. Lutter L: Pronation biomechanics in runners. Contemp Orthop 2:579–583, 1980.
53. Mack RP: Ankle injuries in athletics. Clin Sports Med 1:71–79, 1982.
54. MacKean LC, Bell G, Burnham RS: Prophylactic ankle bracing vs. taping: Effects on functional performance in female basketball players. J Orthop Sports Phys Ther 22(2):77–81, 1995.
55. Mayhew JL: Effects of ankle taping on motor performance. Athletic Training 7:10–11, 1972.
56. McConnell J: The management of chondromalacia patellae: A long term solution. Aust J Physiother 32:215–223, 1986.
57. Morehouse CA: Evaluation of knee abduction and adduction: The effects of selected exercise programs on knee stability and its relationship to knee injuries in college football. Project report. University Park, PA, Pennsylvania State University, May 1970.
58. Moss CL: Ankle taping: The 8-stirrup technique. Athletic Training 24(4):339–341, 1989.
59. Moss CL, Gorton B, Deter S: A comparison of prescribed rigid orthotic devices and athletic taping support used to modify pronation in runners. J Sport Rehab 2:179–188, 1993.
60. Myburgh KH, Baughan CL, Isaacs SK: The effects of ankle guards and taping on joint motion before, during and after a squash match. Am J Sports Med 12:441–446, 1984.
61. Nawoczenski DA, Cook TM, Saltman CL: The effect of foot orthotics on three dimensional kinematics of the leg and rearfoot during running. J Orthop Sports Phys Ther 21(6):317–326, 1995.

62. Ottaviani RA, Ashton-Miller JA, Kothari SU, et al: Basketball shoe height and the maximal muscular resistance to applied ankle inversion and eversion moments. Am J Sports Med 23(4):418–423, 1995.

63. Paris DL: The effects of the Swede-O, New Cross and McDavid ankle braces and adhesive ankle taping on speed, balance, agility, and vertical leap. J Athletic Training 27(3):253–256, 1992.

64. Paris DL: The effects of adhesive ankle taping and cloth ankle wrapping on speed, agility, balance and power. Bull Sports Med Sect APTA 44A:1183–1190, 1978.

65. Passerallo AJ, Calabrese GJ: Improving traditional ankle taping techniques with rigid strapping tape. J Athletic Training 29(1):76–77, 1994.

66. Perlau R, Frank C, Fick G: The effect of elastic bandages on human knee proprioception in the uninjured population. Am J Sports Med 23(2):251–255, 1995.

67. Pope MH, Renstrom P, Donnermeyer D, et al: A comparison of ankle taping methods. Med Sci Sports Exerc 19(2):143–147, 1987.

68. Rarick GL, Bigley GK, Ralph MR: The measurable support of the ankle joint by conventional methods of taping. J Bone Joint Surg 44A:1183–1190, 1962.

69. Robinson JR, Frederick EC, Cooper LB: Systematic ankle stabilization and the effect on performance. Med Sci Sports Exerc 18:625–628, 1986.

70. Rovere GD, Clarke TJ, Yates CS, et al: Retrospective comparison of taping and ankle stabilizers in preventing ankle injuries. Am J Sports Med 16(3):228–233, 1988.

71. Rovere GD, Curl WW, Browning DG: Bracing and taping in an office sports medicine practice. Clin Sports Med 8(3):497–515, 1989.

72. Sammacaro J: How I manage turf toe. Physician Sportsmed 16(9):113–118, 1988.

73. Scheuffelen C, Gollhofera A, Lohrer H: Novel functional studies of the stabilizing behavior of ankle joint orthoses. Sportverletz Sportschaden 7(1):30–36, 1993.

74. Schroeder JK: Support for strained and subluxing peroneal tendons. Athletic Training 23(1):45, 66, 1988.

75. Scranton PE, PeDegana LR, Whitesel JP: Gait analysis alterations in support phase forces using supportive devices. Am J Sports Med 10(1):6–11, 1982.

76. Shapiro MS, Kabo JM, Mitchell PN, et al: Ankle sprain prophylaxis: An analysis of the stabilizing effects of braces and tape. Am J Sports Med 22:78–82, 1994.

77. Sims D, Marke JM: Bubble packing: An alternative technique for padding severe thigh contusions. Athletic Training 25(2):163–165, 1990.

78. Sprigings EJ, Pelton JD: An EMG analysis of the effectiveness of external ankle support during sudden ankle inversion. Can J Appl Sport Sci 6:72–75, 1981.

79. Thomas JR, Cotten DJ: Does ankle taping slow down athletes? Coach Athlete 34(4):20, 37, 1977.

80. Thompson K: The effects of ankle taping on static and dynamic balance. Phys Ther 64(5):726–727, 1984.

81. Tropp H, Askling C, Gillquist J: Prevention of ankle sprains. Am J Sports Med 13:259–262, 1985.

82. Tropp H, Ekstrand J, Gillquist J: Factors affecting stabilometry recordings of single leg stance. Am J Sports Med 12(3):185–188, 1984.

83. Vaes P, DeBoeck H, Handelberg F, et al: Comparative radiologic study of the influence of ankle bandages on ankle instability. Am J Sports Med 13:46–50, 1985.

84. Van Dam R, Ruhling RO: Tape composition and performance. Athletic Training JNATA 10:214–216, 1975.

85. Whitesel J, Newell SG: Modified low-dye strapping. Physician Sportsmed 8(9):129, 1980.

86. Wilkerson GB: Comparative biomechanical effects of the standard method of ankle taping and taping method designed to enhance subtalar stability. Am J Sports Med 19:588–595, 1991.

87. Wilkins DR: Taping the subluxing peroneal tendon. Athletic Training 26(4):370–371, 1991.

88. Zylks DR: Alternative taping for plantar fasciitis. Athletic Training 22(4):317–318, 1987.

Use of Orthoses for the Adult with Neurologic Involvement

CYNTHIA M. ZABLOTNY

Adults with neurologic involvement as a result of a cerebrovascular accident, traumatic brain injury, spinal cord injury, or other diagnosis frequently experience problems meeting the functional demands of gait and other related upright activities. An orthosis may be indicated to assist in joint or limb segment realignment, stabilization, or controlled mobility. A thoughtfully prescribed orthosis enables the adult with neurologic involvement to access more efficient movement patterns, to expand his or her repertoire of movement options, and ultimately to reduce the residual gait disability.

The purpose of this chapter is to discuss the role of various lower-limb orthoses in managing some of the common gait deviations displayed by the adult with neurologic involvement. Primary emphasis is on the more commonly prescribed lower-limb braces, although a discussion of the knee-ankle-foot orthosis is also included. The goals of orthotic prescription are addressed as they relate to the biomechanical alterations of human movement in upright function. Normal gait is reviewed at the outset so that a frame of reference exists for subsequent discussion of pathomechanics.

CHALLENGES OF FUNCTION IN UPRIGHT POSTURE DURING GAIT

Understanding the biomechanics of normal gait helps us to appreciate the demands of walking and the continuous challenges to stay upright and to reach our destination in an efficient manner. A working knowledge of the normal gait cycle and its functional tasks, subphases, and critical events is essential before any type of treatment interventions can be introduced. The terminology used to describe gait in this chapter is based on the Rancho Los Amigos Medical Center Observational Gait Analysis model, which was developed under the direction of Dr. Jacquelin Perry.[19, 20]

Three basic functional tasks are essential for efficient and successful ambulation. These tasks have been defined as weight acceptance, single-limb support, and swing limb advancement.[19, 20] As its name implies, the first task involves the ability to accept weight onto a forward limb. For this to happen in a smooth manner, this limb must be stable and must be able to absorb the impact of superincumbent body weight. At the same time, forward progression of the limb and the body must be initiated. The task of single-limb support involves the ability of the body to continue forward progression over the weight-bearing limb, a task that requires stability over a reduced base of support. Lastly, swing limb advancement involves unweighting of the limb, followed by its forward progression until the next step is initiated. Limb clearance is an essential component of this functional task of swing limb advancement.

Although limb movement during gait involves multisegment motion, some movements clearly take precedence in their importance and their contribu-

TABLE 8–1
Normal Gait Cycle*

Functional Task	Gait Subphase	Critical Events
Weight acceptance	Initial contact	Heel-first contact
	Loading response	Hip stability
		Controlled knee flexion to 15 degrees
		Ankle plantarflexion to 10 degrees
Single-limb support	Midstance	Controlled tibial advancement
	Terminal stance	Ankle locked in 10 degrees of dorsiflexion
		Heel rise
		Trailing limb posture
Swing limb advancement	Preswing	Passive knee flexion to 40 degrees
	Initial swing	Hip flexion to 15 degrees
		Knee flexion to 60 degrees
	Midswing	Continued hip flexion to 25 degrees
		Ankle dorsiflexion to 0 degrees
	Terminal swing	Knee extension to neutral

*The normal gait cycle is divided into three functional tasks and eight corresponding gait subphases. The contribution of the critical events of each subphase is discussed in the text.

Adapted from Rancho Los Amigos Medical Center, Physical Therapy Department and Pathokinesiology Laboratory, Observational Gait Analysis Handbook, LAREI, Inc., Downey, CA, 1993. Used with permission.

tion to the ultimate goal of completing all three of the functional tasks of gait. The Rancho system refers to such movements as the critical events of the gait cycle.[19, 20] These events are summarized in Table 8–1 and are elaborated as each of the gait subphases is subsequently discussed.

Weight Acceptance

Initial contact is described as the moment when the foot touches the ground. In normal gait, this contact is made with the heel first. The limb is outstretched in front of the body as contact is made, with the hip in approximately 25 degrees of hip flexion, while the knee and ankle retain neutral joint alignment. The ground-reaction force at initial contact lies posterior to the ankle joint axis, creating a plantarflexion moment.[25] This ground-reaction force also causes eversion at the subtalar joint, an event that assists with shock absorption. During loading response, the foot reacts to the plantarflexion moment with a 10-degree plantarflexion response that is controlled eccentrically by the pretibial musculature, which includes the anterior tibialis, extensor digitorum longus, and extensor hallucis longus. As the foot is brought down to the ground, forward tibial advancement is initiated. The knee responds to this tibial progression by flexing to approximately 15 degrees. This motion assists in absorbing the shock of weight acceptance but presents a challenge to knee stability as a result of the posture that is assumed. An eccentric response by the quadriceps is essential at this subphase to maintain the required knee stability. Hip stability must be maintained during loading, a task that demands an active response of the hip extensor musculature. The challenges to hip stability are great at this point in the gait cycle. Body weight is accepted onto a hip that is already positioned in 25 degrees of flexion. Both the forward momentum of the trunk and the hip flexion torque created as a result of the location of the ground-reaction force vector have a destabilizing effect on the hip. The response of the hip extensor muscles enables the maintenance of an upright trunk posture and prevents further hip flexion.

Single-Limb Support

As the body moves into single-limb support, stability and forward progression continue to be a requirement. During the first single-limb support subphase, defined as midstance, the body progresses forward over a foot that remains in full contact with the ground. As body weight moves anteriorly, the tibia shows a controlled advancement to a position of approximately 5 degrees of dorsiflexion. The soleus muscle initiates the restraint of the tibia, followed by the gastrocnemius once the knee reaches an extended posture. This control of the tibia is critical at this point because it enables the knee and ultimately the hip to achieve alignments that favor stability. Once the ground-reaction force vector passes anterior to the knee joint axis, the knee can maintain its extended posture without additional quadriceps activity.[25] Hip extension to a neutral position is facilitated by the momentum generated by the contralateral swing limb. Frontal plane stability is essential during midstance and is achieved through the action of the hip abductors.

During the next single-limb support subphase, defined as terminal stance, the body advances forward ahead of the foot. To accomplish this task, continued eccentric plantarflexion muscle control is required to counter the large dorsiflexion torque created by body weight. By the end of terminal stance, the ankle is essentially locked in a position of 10 degrees of dorsiflexion as body weight progresses over the forefoot and the heel begins to rise. These events contribute to a normal step length on the contralateral limb. As a result of the forward progression of the body, the stance limb assumes a trailing position with respect to the trunk. The hip assumes a hyperextended posture, while the knee remains fully extended. Body alignment ensures the stability of these joints without the need for additional muscle activity.

Swing Limb Advancement

The functional task of swing limb advancement begins with the subphase of preswing, which is defined as a period of double-limb support in which the stance limb is rapidly unloaded and prepared for swing. As body weight progresses forward, only the metatarsals remain in contact with the ground on the preswing limb. As the transfer of body weight occurs from one limb to the next, the ankle plantarflexes 20 degrees, and the knee passively moves into 40 degrees of flexion, an event facilitated by the previous attainment of a trailing limb posture and the forward progression of body weight. Attaining 40 degrees of knee flexion is a critical event in gait, in that it prepares the limb for initial swing. During preswing, the thigh moves forward to a neutral position as the limb is unweighted, and the tibia advances anteriorly.

The next subphase of initial swing involves a period of thigh advancement during which the foot clears the ground. The forward momentum of the thigh that began in preswing is now augmented by an active hip flexor response to ensure advancement to 15 degrees of hip flexion. Foot clearance is achieved as a result of the knee's flexing to 60 degrees, an event that is critical to the dynamics of normal gait. Successful attainment of the required knee flexion in initial swing results from a critically timed combination of proper preswing knee flexion, momentum from the thigh's quick advancement, and an active muscle response by the short head of the biceps femoris. The 10-degree plantarflexed ankle position in initial swing does not contribute to limb clearance.

Thigh advancement continues into the next gait subphase of midswing until the hip reaches a position of 25 degrees of flexion. This additional hip flexion occurs as a result of the thigh's momentum generated in initial swing. The knee begins to extend forward, reaching a vertical tibial alignment that corresponds to a position of 25 degrees of flexion. Thigh advancement in midswing occurs passively in response to the hip flexion momentum generated in initial swing. Foot clearance in midswing is due to the action of the pretibial muscles as they dorsiflex the ankle to neutral.

Terminal swing, a transitional subphase of gait, refers to the time when the limb achieves its maximal forward reach. Some of the events that occur in terminal swing actually assist the limb in preparing for the onset of weight acceptance. Hip flexion beyond 25 degrees is curtailed through the action of the long hamstring muscles, which serve to decelerate the thigh. Knee extension is achieved as a result of an active quadriceps response. The ankle continues to maintain its neutral position through the action of the pretibial muscles. This position prepares the foot for a heel-first initial contact. The motions of hip flexion, knee extension, and 5 degrees of transverse plane forward rotation of the pelvis contribute to the step length capabilities of this forward limb. An additional contribution to step length is made by the contralateral stance limb as it concurrently meets the challenges of body weight progression over the forefoot in terminal stance.

CHALLENGES OF FUNCTION IN UPRIGHT POSTURE FOR ADULTS WITH NEUROLOGIC INVOLVEMENT

An individual with an intact nervous system can readily meet the demands of gait in an efficient manner. For the adult with neurologic involvement, however, each functional task of gait presents a unique challenge to that person's need to maintain stability while still progressing forward. Some of these problems lend themselves to orthotic remediation, whereas others are not significantly improved by the use of an orthosis.

The first step in determining appropriate treatment strategies requires a comprehensive movement analysis. To realize the full impact and scope of movement deficits, it is helpful to perform an analysis across a range of walking speeds, distances, and terrains. By combining knowledge of the normal components of gait at each specific subphase with a consideration of the patient's motor control and balance, joint mobility, proprioception, and perceptual skills, the health care provider can identify the primary gait deficits and the variables that might contribute to their appearance. An appropriate decision regarding the need for orthotic intervention can then be made.

The purpose of the following discussion is to present some of the more common gait deviations that are demonstrated by the adult with neurologic involvement. Given the complexity and the wide range of problems experienced by this population, the deviations listed here are not intended to be all-inclusive. The discussion focuses primarily on the impact of specific gait deviations in the sagittal plane. The clinician should recognize that the combination of movement deficits a patient experiences will affect his or her capabilities in all three planes of motion. It is equally important for the clinician to realize the interdependence that exists among the three functional tasks of gait and the significant impact of a deficit in one task on the sequence of movements in subsequent functional tasks. Likewise, the interrelationship of one limb to the other must always be considered. A problem in weight acceptance or single-limb support on one limb impacts the swing limb capabilities of the opposite limb.

Weight Acceptance

During weight acceptance, it is common for the adult with neurologic involvement to display alignments throughout the lower extremity and trunk that promote stability at the expense of mobility or forward progression. The ensuing alignments are predictable and depend on the manner of initial contact demonstrated by the patient. For example, a forefoot initial contact sets up a chain of events in the stance limb that precludes adequate tibial advancement and minimizes the shock-absorbing effect normally provided by subtalar joint eversion and knee flexion during limb loading. As the patient attempts to bring the foot down to the ground following a forefoot-first initial contact, the tibia is thrust posteriorly, resulting in a weight-bearing position involving excessive ankle plantarflexion and subtalar inversion. Proximally, the knee assumes an extended posture, the hip is flexed with respect to a vertical alignment, and the trunk is brought forward (Fig. 8–1). This weight-bearing posture results in a ground-reaction force

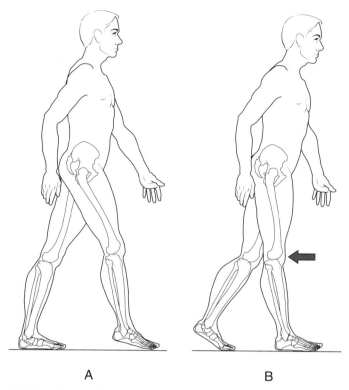

FIGURE 8–1. *A*, Knee and ankle joint kinematics are altered as a result of a forefoot-first initial contact. *B*, The tibia moves posteriorly as the foot is brought down to the ground, causing a knee extension moment to occur as the limb is loaded.

vector at loading response that is anterior to the ankle and knee, thereby reducing the normal plantarflexion and knee flexion moments.[2] A patient choosing this movement option may feel that the forward limb is more secure and less likely to buckle. This strategy, however, does not facilitate the tibial advancement needed to get the body moving in a forward direction.

The weight acceptance strategy described may be seen in a patient with various impairments, such as reduced dynamic knee extension control, delayed timing or weakness of the eccentric pretibial response, premature activation of the soleus response, the presence of plantarflexion or equinovarus contractures, or impaired proprioception at the knee or ankle.[19, 20]

An alternative pattern of limb response that might be demonstrated in weight acceptance consists of excessive hip and knee flexion, resulting in a highly unstable limb (Fig. 8–2). This response is frequently seen in the patient who has trunk, hip, and knee extensor weakness and who is unable to demonstrate adequate eccentric control as body weight is loaded onto the limb. The presence of hip or knee flexion contractures may also predispose the limb to this movement pattern.[19, 20]

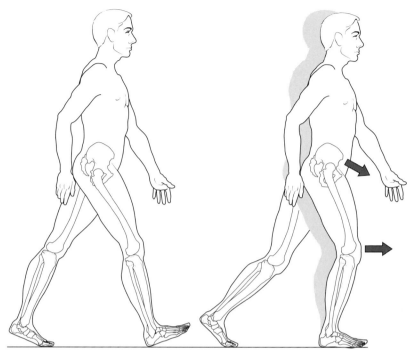

FIGURE 8-2. Proximal weakness during weight acceptance results in a rapid acceleration of the tibia in the line of progression. This pattern causes excessive hip and knee flexion *(arrows)* and a highly unstable period of weight acceptance.

Single-Limb Support

The weight acceptance strategy involving excessive ankle plantarflexion and an extended knee posture is often maintained as the patient moves into the single-limb support subphases. The inherent stability that is gained from these malalignments may become increasingly important as the base of support decreases from two limbs to just a single limb. As the patient moves into single-limb support, it often becomes increasingly difficult to progress over and then ahead of the supporting foot because this chosen movement strategy does not allow the patient to readily access the necessary range of ankle dorsiflexion (Fig. 8–3). As a result, progression over the forefoot is limited, as is contralateral step length.[10] A secondary gain from persisting in the posture of excessive plantarflexion with the heel still held on the ground is that the plantar support surface is larger than it would be if a heel-off posture and progression onto the forefoot occurred. From a biomechanical standpoint, the ability to progress over the foot in single-limb support and to achieve a trailing limb posture requires the presence of adequate hindfoot, midfoot, and forefoot range of motion, as well as adequate hip, knee, and lumbar extension range of motion. Difficulty achieving these critical events

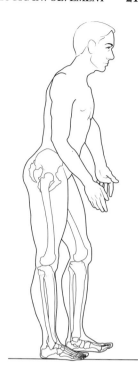

FIGURE 8–3. Excessive plantarflexion in midstance limits forward tibial progression. Lack of a heel rise in terminal stance prevents adequate body progression over the stance limb and results in a reduction in the length of the contralateral step.

may be a result of range-of-motion impairments in these areas. Compensation for weak plantarflexors or weak knee extensors may also promote the maintenance of this posture of excessive plantarflexion, knee extension, or hyperextension (if available) with a forward trunk lean.[19, 20]

An alternative alignment that may be seen in the adult patient may involve excessive hip and knee flexion in combination with excessive ankle dorsiflexion (Fig. 8–4). The trunk may maintain a vertical alignment over the flexed limb, provided that the patient has an adequate lumbar lordosis. More often, the trunk is inclined forward with respect to the vertical because the patient may not have enough lumbar extension range of motion to assume an erect posture over the flexed lower extremity. Although the tibial segment is already inclined forward when this limb posture is adopted, the benefits of controlled tibial advancement in combination with an extended hip and knee position are not attained, resulting in another situation that limits the achievement of a trailing limb position in preparation for swing limb advancement.

An excessively flexed limb may result from either distal or proximal control problems, or a combination of both. Excessive tibial progression in single-limb support is frequently caused by an uncompensated calf weakness. The knee and hip assume a flexed posture as the patient attempts realignment over the base of support. Proximal instability due to trunk or hip

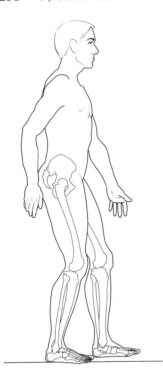

FIGURE 8-4. Excessive ankle dorsiflexion is frequently accompanied by excessive hip and knee flexion and a flat foot posture throughout all single-limb support. Contralateral step length is reduced. The swing limb is brought closer to the ground, presenting a challenge to the task of foot clearance.

extensor weakness may preclude a patient's ability to achieve a vertical femoral or trunk alignment, especially in early midstance. Again, a flexed posture is likely to be adopted at the ankle as a compensation for the proximal instability. Inadequate knee or hip extension range of motion may also be primary causes of this malalignment into flexion. This limb posture places the ground-reaction force vector anterior to the hip joint and posterior to the knee joint, increasing the extensor muscle requirements at these joints. For the adult patient with lower-limb extensor weakness involving the hip, knee, or ankle, this is a difficult posture to assume and to function within efficiently. An additional problem faced by the patient in excessive stance limb flexion is potential difficulty in clearing the contralateral swing limb, which has been relatively lengthened as a result of the stance limb malalignments. Because many adult patients have bilateral involvement as a result of their primary neurologic disorder or as a result of secondary medical problems such as diabetes, this interaction of limb function is an important point to consider in identifying the causes of their gait dysfunction.

Frontal plane instability, as a result of abductor weakness, is most notably observed during single-limb stance. Instability in this plane of movement may contribute to impaired balance. Additionally, a severe contralateral pelvic drop that is not compensated by a lateral trunk lean over the stance

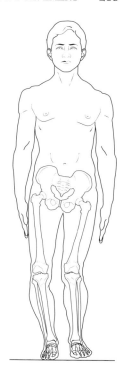

FIGURE 8–5. An uncompensated pelvic drop in single-limb support increases the varus moments at the hip, knee, and ankle of the stance limb. Single-limb balance and stability are challenged by the sudden downward displacement of body weight as the pelvis drops. The reduced base of support that results from the varus attitude of the subtalar joint further reduces stability.

limb may result in a relatively adducted thigh position on the stance limb. This position frequently reduces the patient's base of support from the whole foot to the lateral border only, resulting in a varus attitude of the foot that is frequently accompanied by plantarflexion (Fig. 8–5).

Swing Limb Advancement

Regardless of whether the single-limb support pattern involves excessive plantarflexion or excessive ankle dorsiflexion, tibial forward progression does not take place in a controlled manner. The persistence of stance phase alignments that interfere with this important event significantly limits a patient's ability to meet the functional demands of swing limb advancement in time. Identification of this interrelationship among the postures assumed in stance and subsequent swing mobility requirements is important not only for patient analysis but also for directing the focus of the physical therapy treatment plan, particularly in the prescription of an orthosis.

As previously outlined, the patient with neurologic involvement may not achieve a heel-off posture or trailing limb position by the completion of terminal stance. The functional implication is that the stance limb is clearly not in a position to be easily unweighted or set up for preswing flexion. As a result, knee flexion remains limited by the end of preswing, and thigh advancement does not begin until initial swing. The delayed timing of this event requires increased hip flexor activity to advance the femur forward quickly. The patient with neurologic involvement frequently cannot meet this requirement because of impaired timing or decreased strength of the hip flexor muscles. Limb clearance, especially in initial swing, may not be achieved as a result of the limitations experienced in knee flexion range of motion and the problems noted with thigh advancement. The inadequate forward momentum that is so crucial to the achievement of adequate knee flexion places the knee flexors at a disadvantage as more torque is required to clear the foot. A toe drag is a common deviation seen in many patients, resulting in safety concerns during ambulation (Fig. 8–6).

Limb clearance is accomplished more easily in midswing than in initial swing. The momentum generated from the thigh advancement in initial swing contributes to this clearance in midswing. Limb clearance problems may persist if there is restricted hip motion or if the patient is not able to obtain a neutral ankle angle.

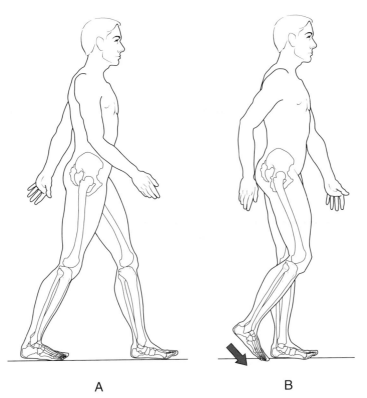

A   B

FIGURE 8–6. *A,* Limited progression over the stance limb results in inadequate knee flexion in preswing. *B,* Continued limitations in initial-swing knee flexion interfere with foot clearance, resulting in a toe drag and a potential loss of balance.

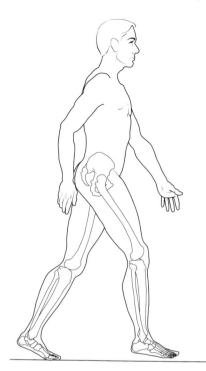

FIGURE 8-7. Excessive ankle plantarflexion in terminal swing prevents the attainment of a heel-first initial contact and predisposes the patient to limb segment alignments that discourage forward progression in weight acceptance.

Difficulties maintaining a neutral ankle position in terminal swing are common in this patient population, resulting in an ankle that is excessively plantarflexed by the end of terminal swing. Adequate forward reach of the swing limb is frequently not attained because motor control deficits do not promote the required combined movements of forward pelvic rotation in the transverse plane, hip flexion, and knee extension (Fig. 8–7). As a result of these inadequate terminal swing postures, the patient is set up to make floor contact with the forefoot first or with the entire foot, and the whole pattern of stance phase malalignments is once again initiated.

GOALS OF ORTHOTIC INTERVENTION

As illustrated in the discussion of pathomechanics, alignment variations at one segment of the body during gait frequently alter the movement patterns throughout the entire lower limb and trunk. It follows, then, that the goals of orthotic prescription should address this relationship among body segments. These goals represent a departure, perhaps, from a more traditional approach to orthotic prescription that focuses on remediating a specific single-joint problem and that places less emphasis on the ramifications of this treatment for whole-body upright function.

The goal of orthotic prescription in the adult neurologic patient is to alter the components of movement, as outlined by Fisher and Yakura,[7] that contribute to the fluidity and versatility of gait. These essential movement components are interrelated and include the base of support, alignment, sequencing, and issues of stability and mobility. Although an orthotic intervention may primarily be aimed at altering one of these components, benefits are frequently realized among the others also.

Biomechanical Considerations in Orthotic Prescription

REESTABLISHING AN APPROPRIATE BASE OF SUPPORT. Body progression in normal gait takes place over a constantly changing base of support. The specific plantar surface area of the foot that is in contact with the ground at any single point in the gait cycle directly influences lower-extremity joint kinematics and closed-chain kinetic responses. Clinically, a reduction in appropriate foot contact area at a given point in the gait cycle may result in stance limb instability, high localized pressures, or an inability to progress efficiently over the base of support.

An orthosis may assist in achieving and in maintaining an appropriate base of support during critical moments in stance. Appropriate adjustments in the base of support may enhance single- and double-limb balance, single-limb support time on the side of orthotic application, contralateral step length, and foot pressure distribution. These adjustments, in turn, lead to availability of a broader range of movement options throughout the foot and the entire closed kinematic chain. The patient has the potential to be a more versatile, functional ambulator if all these secondary benefits of orthotic intervention are realized. To illustrate this point, consider the patient who initially contacts the ground with the lateral border of the entire foot and maintains this varus attitude throughout midstance. During initial contact, the primary goal of the orthosis is to reestablish the heel as the appropriate base of support. Achievement of this goal facilitates a successful transition into flat foot and enhances the patient's ability to move the tibia anteriorly. Another benefit of reestablishing the heel as the initial base of support is that it facilitates an eversion response at the subtalar joint and a flexion response at the knee during weight acceptance, both of which contribute to shock absorption. The orthotic goal in midstance is to maintain the entire foot in a weight-bearing position. This position assists with pressure distribution and with maximizing the base of support so that single-limb balance is enhanced. The patient is more likely to progress the tibia anteriorly and to move into the appropriate dorsiflexed ankle position if weight is borne across the entire foot.

CONTROLLING RATE, EXCURSION, AND DIRECTION OF SEGMENTAL MOVEMENT. Another goal of orthotic application may be directed at controlling the rate, excursion, or direction of the foot and the tibial and femoral segments during weight acceptance and continuing into single-limb support. Achieving this goal promotes improved alignment of all the lower-extremity segments and the trunk so that body progression over the stance foot occurs in a manner that is controlled, efficient, and inherently stable. This benefit can be illustrated by considering the use of an orthosis to control excessive and rapidly occurring knee flexion in midstance. An orthosis that limits the range of ankle dorsiflexion and that has design features that control the rate of tibial progression would be indicated in this situation. Providing orthotic control for this deviation enhances limb stability and efficiency by appropriately realigning the ground-reaction force vector over the foot, thereby reducing the muscular requirements on the knee and hip extensors and the ankle plantarflexors. Slowing the rate of tibial progression with an orthosis also reduces the rate of femoral advancement. This realignment facilitates controlled advancement of the body over the base of support.

IMPROVING ENERGY EFFICIENCY. A third goal of orthotic intervention in stance might be to assist the patient in achieving and in maintaining postures that require less overall metabolic energy expenditure or that reduce the demand for a specific muscular response.[30] This goal is of particular importance when addressing the management of the patient with progressive weakness or the client exhibiting a stable pattern of weakness accompanied by changes in body weight, joint disease, or other concerns. Directing attention to goals concerning energy efficiency may affect the short- and long-term functional outcomes of the gait disability a patient experiences. Reducing the energy requirements of ambulation with the use of an orthosis may enable the household ambulator to meet the endurance and speed requirements of walking in the community.

An orthosis can assist a patient in achieving and in maintaining limb postures that promote energy-efficient alignments and reduce muscular demand. A secondary benefit of enhanced alignment is that segmental momentum can be optimized, a situation that further reduces the need for any additional muscular response.[20]

POSITIONING THE FOOT FOR CLEARANCE AND WEIGHT ACCEPTANCE. It is not uncommon for the patient with neurologic involvement to experience problems managing both the stance and the swing phases of gait. There are some instances when isolated weakness interferes with swing limb advancement only. Regardless of the situation, the goals of orthotic intervention in swing are primarily focused on optimally positioning the foot to clear the floor during limb advancement and on achieving a heel-first initial contact.[28] If successfully achieved, the first of these goals improves patient safety by eliminating a toe drag and potential loss of balance. A more energy-efficient gait pattern may be adopted once limb clearance is achieved because compensatory gait deviations, such as excessive hip and knee flexion, a lateral trunk lean, excessive hip abduction or rotation, or contralateral vaulting, are minimized or eliminated. Additionally, the ability to make contact with the heel first, as opposed to a flat foot or forefoot-first initial contact, helps to facilitate forward tibial advancement once stance is initiated. This ability is optimized in brace designs that encourage flexibility into subtalar eversion so that weight can be borne on the heel.

Neurologic Considerations in Orthotic Prescription

The goals of orthotic prescription previously outlined focus on improving the biomechanics of gait. In the literature addressing orthotic use in the population of adults with central nervous system dysfunction, several authors discuss the effects of bracing on the input and the output of the nervous system itself.[4, 14, 18, 23, 26, 32] Realignment or support of any segment of the body through the use of an orthosis results in alterations in the proprioceptive and tactile input to the central nervous system. This claim is certainly straightforward and irrefutable. Problems arise, however, when one is speculating how an orthosis might alter the output of the central nervous system. Certain orthotic designs have been purported to reduce tone or to stimulate tonic reflexes in the foot, which in turn may inhibit abnormal foot postures.[4, 14, 18, 23, 26, 32] Suggestions have been made as to the neurophysiologic principles that might explain such phenomena, if in fact they do occur, but to date no clear evidence supports the notion that an alteration in the output of the central nervous system will occur as a result of a specific orthotic design.[4]

Further research is needed to lend support to the empirical claims suggesting an inhibition of excessive muscle tone with an orthosis. These research efforts need to address the effects of orthotic biomechanical realignment on both the peripheral and the central processing phenomena that control muscle tone and movement. Documentation of such evidence presents a distinct challenge, as currently there is no widely accepted reliable and valid method to describe tone, especially as it correlates with active limb movement and overall function.[9] Quantitative assessments of kinematic or kinetic variables with specific orthotic designs may help identify and document changes in movement patterns and may clarify the neurophysiologic processes that underlie these changes.[1, 11]

ANKLE-FOOT ORTHOSES: DESIGN AND COMPONENTS

A wide range of ankle-foot orthosis (AFO) designs are used in managing the adult patient with neurologic involvement. These designs vary regionally and frequently reflect the preferences of those orthotists involved with their fabrication. As members of the rehabilitation team, the physician, the physical therapist, and the orthotist each plays a role in educating the patient in the decision-making process involving orthotic prescription. Team members assume responsibility for identifying any potential benefits of a specific orthosis, as well as the limitations its use might impose on the patient as a variety of functional tasks are performed. The prescriptive process is a dynamic one, especially in this population of patients. As a result, the patient should know that alternative orthoses might be indicated as individual needs change. The rehabilitation team bears the responsibility for educating the patient and the family about the costs involved with orthotic prescription, and they must assist the patient in making a prescriptive decision that considers all these factors.

It is frequently difficult to remain informed of the changing designs of lower-extremity bracing. Collaboration with the orthotist is the best way to become educated regarding new design possibilities and fabrication materials. Regardless of the choice of orthotic design or fabrication materials, the clinician needs to make an educated decision about whether a particular brace will meet the needs of the patient. A logical assessment of some of the key characteristics of a proposed bracing design and its fabrication materials will enable the clinician to decide if a specific brace is indeed the right choice for the patient (Table 8–2).

TABLE 8–2
Essential Features of AFOs: Consideration of Their Impact on Biomechanics of Gait

Features of AFO	Impact on Gait Biomechanics
Length of the foot segment	Affects the length of the lever arm of the foot; as this is reduced, tibial restraint is lessened
	Support of the foot increases as this segment length increases, resulting in a greater ability to affect multiple joint alignments in the foot and lower extremity
Rigidity of the foot-ankle area	Flexibility facilitates closed kinematic chain movements at multiple segments; stiffness promotes a more stabilizing effect at the expense of movement
	Rigidity is influenced by the inherent characteristics of material, thickness of material, and position of trim lines with respect to anatomic ankle axis
Relationship of brace height to tibial height	More direct control of tibial sagittal plane movement is available as the brace height approximates tibial height
Stiffness of the material used as an upright	As the material becomes stiffer, tibial movement becomes more constrained
Multiplanar alignment of the brace with respect to the patient's anatomic alignment	Enhances effectiveness of AFO design to promote flexibility or stability; malalignment may result in undesired effects such as excessive mobility at a specific foot or lower-extremity joint

The capabilities of any AFO depend on the relative contribution of each of the essential design features outlined in Table 8–2 that dictate where body segment restraint or mobility will occur. These AFO characteristics have an impact on the biomechanics of gait because of their ability to influence joint mobility and ground-reaction forces. The interaction of these design features is important to consider. For example, even though a brace may be very rigid in the area of the ankle joint, its ability to restrain the tibia may be severely reduced if it is only of supramalleolar height. If the goal of an AFO is to control the rate and direction of tibial advancement and to reestablish an adequate base of support in stance, then the brace must be able to meet the various torque demands placed on it by superincumbent body weight. Such demands require the use of more rigid orthotic materials and a relatively increased brace height with respect to tibial height. The job of the swing-phase–control orthosis is a more simple one, in that its primary goal is to support the weight of the foot and shoe, approximately 2 pounds.[16]

Footwear choices have an impact on the dynamic response of any orthotic design. Alterations in footwear features, such as heel design and height, sole material, or angle of the toe taper, can directly affect the forces involved with walking or the time during which these forces may act. Decisions regarding footwear should be made with the orthotic prescription in mind so that each component may complement the effectiveness of the other.

Types of Ankle-Foot Orthoses and Indications for Their Prescription

The following bracing designs are capable of providing some degree of control during stance, swing, or both phases of gait. These bracing designs are presented in descending order, from those braces providing the most rigid ankle control to those providing the least amount of control. Included are designs considered to be traditional AFO offerings. The advantages and disadvantages of these AFOs are reviewed. Information on some of the newer bracing designs and orthotic inserts is provided at the completion of this section.

RIGID POLYPROPYLENE AFO. The custom-molded rigid polypropylene AFO is indicated when maximal tibial restraint is required to prevent either excessive ankle dorsiflexion or plantarflexion from occurring in stance (Fig. 8–8). This bracing design is also indicated to control mediolateral instability at the subtalar joint during stance.[17, 29] An additional benefit of this AFO is that it helps to facilitate limb clearance in midswing and positions the foot in terminal swing for a heel-first initial contact. A rigid polypropylene AFO can be especially useful for the patient whose upright skills are impaired by both proximal and distal weakness. The application of this AFO decreases the degrees of freedom through which such a patient must have stance control by essentially eliminating ankle joint motion.[17] As a result, initial

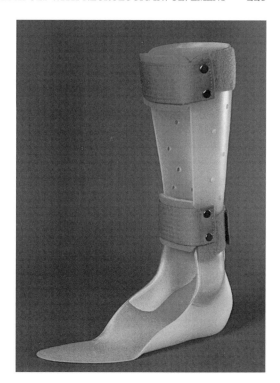

FIGURE 8-8. The rigid polypropylene ankle-foot orthosis (AFO) is capable of providing tibial control in stance. The location of the anterior trim lines, the thickness of the plastic, and the overall height of this brace contribute to its stabilizing abilities.

rehabilitation efforts can be directed toward the development of trunk and hip control over a base of support that is more stable owing to the AFO. This brace offers another advantage to the patient with significant physical impairment, as it is a relatively lightweight design. Other appealing aspects of this AFO include its cosmesis and its ability to be worn within different footwear, provided that a consistent heel height is maintained among different pairs of shoes. Most footwear, if bought to be a half size wider and longer than the foot, will accommodate this brace.

The tibial restraint offered by this AFO presents some disadvantages. Transitional movements that require ankle flexibility are compromised as a result of the rigid structure of this brace. For example, a patient moving from sitting to standing with a rigid polypropylene AFO set at a neutral ankle position is likely to experience difficulty initiating and executing this task as a result of an inability to assume the dorsiflexed ankle position that has been documented as the usual starting condition for this task.[22] To rise with an AFO set at a neutral angle, a patient needs to adopt a new movement strategy that compensates for this mobility restraint. Other functional tasks, such as bending over or climbing stairs, may also be affected by the rigidity of this bracing design. The constraint of this AFO prevents the use of an ankle strategy during upright function and forces the patient to rely on a hip or stepping strategy to maintain balance.[24]

Use of this brace requires that the patient's limb volume remain relatively constant so that adequate fit can be maintained without undue pressure. If the intent of the brace is for postoperative foot positioning following procedures such as a heel cord lengthening, a polypropylene design is not indicated owing to the likelihood of postoperative edema. A metal AFO may be a better choice when limb volume fluctuations are present.

A comprehensive gait analysis must be performed to determine the desired ankle angle before a rigid polypropylene AFO is fabricated.[5] Small changes in this angle may have significant effects on a patient's gait and functional abilities.[10] Whenever possible, the optimal ankle angle is best determined through trial and error with a temporary brace that is adjustable. If this option does not exist, the brace angle should be determined through observational gait analysis and movement analysis across a variety of functional tasks. It is essential to consider the patient's proximal control capabilities when making this decision. A dorsiflexed angle may cause a patient to feel unstable in that it encourages flexion torques at the hip and the knee. A patient who lacks adequate hip and knee extensor control to counter these torques may feel that the brace is causing the limb to collapse rather than making it feel more stable. Conversely, an excessively plantarflexed ankle angle will interfere with the initiation of transitional tasks such as moving from sitting to standing, despite the fact that the patient may feel more stable once in a static standing position. Swing phase limb clearance may also be negatively affected with this plantarflexed ankle setting.

The rigidity of the polypropylene bracing design results from a compilation of the bracing characteristics that have been presented in Table 8–2. A polypropylene thickness of approximately $\frac{3}{16}$ to $\frac{1}{4}$ inch provides enough strength to the foot and ankle region of the brace to control the movement of the tibia in weight acceptance and single-limb support. This thickness of material also provides increased stiffness to the brace as it extends superiorly along the length of the tibia. Upwardly this brace extends to approximately $\frac{3}{4}$ inch below the head of the fibula, a height that assists in achieving maximal tibial restraint. To maximize the rigidity of the foot and ankle region to control the tibia, the anterior trim lines of this brace extend anterior to both malleoli. Lehmann et al[12] identified this particular design feature as having a significant impact on the effectiveness of the brace in controlling the dynamics of terminal stance. The foot plate generally extends at least to the metatarsal heads or to the toes. Altering any or all of these design features has an impact on the overall rigidity of this brace.

BICHANNEL ADJUSTABLE ANKLE LOCKING (BiCAAL) AFO. Another traditional AFO design used primarily to enhance tibial or subtalar joint control in stance is the bichannel adjustable ankle locking (BiCAAL) AFO, also referred to as a double-adjustable ankle joint (DAAJ) AFO (Fig. 8–9).[3, 16, 29] The usefulness of this type of AFO is directly related to the adjustability options of the ankle joint. This brace can be locked at a specific joint angle, or movement can be allowed within a designated ankle range. This flexibility can be advantageous when working with patients with recent neurologic involvement or with those who have a rapidly changing clinical picture. Brace adjustments can be easily made to accommodate changes in a patient's walking abilities.

This type of orthosis can also provide control of the foot during midswing to facilitate foot clearance. Proper foot positioning for terminal swing can also be maintained. Motion within the brace can be a useful option during loading response in some clinical situations. For example, the quick plantarflexion motion that occurs at the ankle following heel strike can be accommodated to help the foot contact the ground and to initiate the forward displacement of the tibia.

Although the adjustability of this bracing design offers a number of clinical advantages, this brace is not for everyone. Major disadvantages of the BiCAAL AFO include its lack of cosmetic appeal and the inability of the wearer to use alternative footwear. The weight of this brace, ranging between 2.5 and 4.0 pounds, can also present a problem for the patient with poor limb advancement capabilities at the hip.

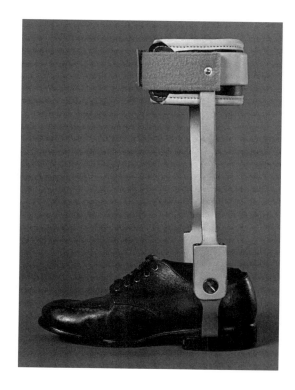

FIGURE 8–9. The bichannel adjustable ankle locking ankle-foot orthosis (BiCAAL AFO) offers a wide range of adjustability options but lacks cosmetic appeal.

This type of AFO provides sagittal and frontal plane movement control through a number of essential design components. The brace consists of two aluminum uprights and a calf band, two double-adjustable ankle joints, and a stainless steel stirrup that attaches the uprights to the shoe[5] (see Fig. 8–9). The calf band, which is usually about 2 inches wide, extends approximately 1 inch below the head of the fibula and fits snugly around the lower leg. If the ankle joint is to be locked during use, the shoe must be equipped with a 1-inch-wide metal shank placed between the leather outer sole and the inner sole. This shank most commonly extends to the metatarsal head area and helps to stiffen the shoe, making it a rigid structure over which the brace uprights can control motion. Inadequate shank length may cause the brace and tibial segment to buckle forward into excessive dorsiflexion in response to the dorsiflexion torque experienced in single-limb support. Shank length can be extended beyond the metatarsal heads if more rigidity is needed in the sole of the shoe.

At times it may be necessary to reinforce the shoe to enable the brace to restrain tibial advancement better in a patient who walks vigorously or who is heavy. The shoe can be reinforced with a heavy-duty stirrup attachment whose base extends $\frac{1}{2}$ inch proximal to the metatarsal head area (Fig. 8–10).[15] An additional layer of sole material is placed over this stirrup attachment to stiffen further the base of support of the shoe and brace combination.

The internal set-up of the ankle joint channels determines the range of

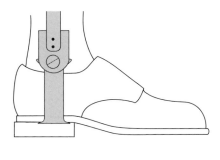

A

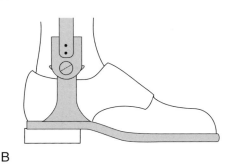

B

FIGURE 8–10. *A,* A conventional stirrup attachment links the brace uprights to the shoe. *B,* A heavy-duty stirrup has a widened base. The rigidity of the brace and shoe is further reinforced by the addition of an extra layer of sole material.

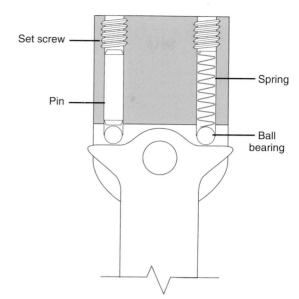

FIGURE 8–11. The internal anatomy of the double-adjustable ankle joint. Ankle joint mobility restrictions result from the location of the pins in the anterior and posterior channels of the orthotic joint. A spring may occupy one of the channels, as depicted here. The ball bearing allows the brace uprights to pivot with ease over the brace stirrup. The set screw can be adjusted easily to change the relative positions of the rods in each of the channels.

movement through which the brace will act. Figure 8–11 depicts the internal anatomy of this double-adjustable ankle joint. Metal rods can be used in the anterior or posterior channels, depending on whether sagittal plane motion restrictions are necessary as the patient moves into dorsiflexion or plantarflexion, respectively.[16] It is also possible to place a spring in the posterior channels to assist with foot clearance during midswing. To achieve the optimal orthotic benefit, the ankle joints should be aligned with the anatomic joint axes, so that the medial joint is slightly anterior to the lateral one. The brace uprights are designed to hug the limb without actually contacting it and are contoured to correspond to the wearer's leg anatomy.

   COMBINED METAL AND PLASTIC DESIGNS. A wide selection of lower-limb bracing designs incorporate a combination of metal and polypropylene components, thus capturing in one device the best features of both the metal AFO and its plastic counterpart. A rigid polypropylene AFO consisting of a foot plate and lower-leg segment connected by double-adjustable ankle joints affords ankle adjustment flexibility with a more cosmetically appealing and lightweight brace design (Fig. 8–12). This type of brace is indicated primarily for stance phase control, although swing phase assistance could also be gained through proper set-up of the ankle joint channels. The foot plate and lower-leg segments of a polypropylene AFO can also be connected by other types of metal joints such as the Gaffney joint. Control of sagittal plane motion is offered to a more limited degree with this joint. In some cases, the two portions of the polypropylene shell may be connected by a large Velcro strap that runs along the posterior aspect of the brace. This strap

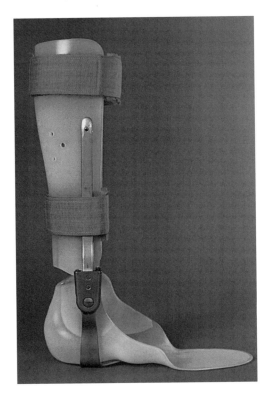

FIGURE 8–12. A rigid polypropylene ankle-foot orthosis (AFO) shell can be modified to incorporate a double-adjustable ankle joint for improved versatility in patient management.

functions as a dorsiflexion stop and can gradually be loosened to allow further dorsiflexion range of motion. Contact between the superior edge of the foot plate shell and the inferior edge of the lower-limb shell acts as a built-in plantarflexion stop.

LIGHTWEIGHT DORSIFLEXION-ASSIST AFO. The lightweight dorsiflexion-assist AFO is designed to assist with foot pick-up, primarily during mid- and terminal swing when ankle dorsiflexion to neutral position is required for adequate limb clearance.[28] The use of this orthosis is not likely to provide limb clearance in initial swing because active knee flexion is the primary event required for the success of this task. This AFO also assists in maintaining good foot positioning in terminal swing so that a heel-first contact is possible. Some minimal mediolateral support in swing is also provided by this brace, in that subtalar joint alignment can be optimized in the presence of mild varus postures.

There are two important differences in the design of this brace when compared with the design of the rigid polypropylene AFO. First, it is lightweight, constructed using $\frac{1}{8}$-inch-thick polypropylene, compared with the $\frac{3}{16}$- to $\frac{1}{4}$-inch-thick polypropylene used for the stance control orthosis. Second, the anterior trim lines fall posterior to the malleoli bilaterally, a feature that further enhances flexibility.[12] These lightweight dorsiflexion AFOs fit and function most effectively when custom-molded, although it is possible to buy prefabricated versions of this orthosis in a limited range of sizes.

FLEXIBLE ANKLE-FOOT ORTHOTIC DESIGNS. Clinicians working with adults with neurologic involvement have recognized the need for patients to progress beyond the limitations imposed by the more traditional AFO offerings. This desire has led to the development of new, progressive AFO designs.[26] It has also created an interest in the application of some specific pediatric orthotic designs to the adult population.[4, 18] Unfortunately, discrepancies exist in the descriptions of some of these designs and in the terminology associated with them, making it difficult to compare functional outcomes among clinicians and authors.[4, 18] To ensure clarity and correctness in orthotic prescription involving these newer bracing designs, the clinician should specify the exact design features required by the patient, rather than referring to the brace only by its name. Such a description should include information such as brace height, trim line position, contour and length of the foot segment, and thickness of material.

DYNAMIC ANKLE-FOOT ORTHOSIS. The dynamic ankle-foot orthosis (DAFO) has been described as a tone-inhibiting orthosis that offers total contact support to the foot and ankle[4, 8, 18] (Fig. 8–13). The intent of the DAFO is to provide improved biomechanical alignment of the foot during stance in order to decrease hypertonia and to control equinovarus or toe-clawing postures.[8, 18] The success of this brace in actually altering or in inhibiting hypertonia remains unproven. Of the two separate single-subject studies, each of which examined the effectiveness of the DAFO in managing the gait deviations of

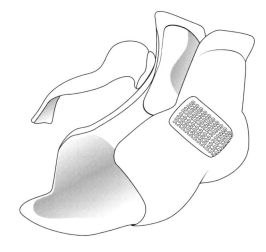

FIGURE 8–13. The dynamic ankle-foot orthosis (DAFO) is a flexible polypropylene brace designed to optimize subtalar joint alignment through its supramalleolar design. (Redrawn from Physical Therapy. Knutson LM, Clark DE. Orthotic devices for ambulation in children with cerebral palsy and myelomeningocele. Phys Ther 71[12]:953, 1991. With the permission of the APTA.)

an adult with neurologic involvement, neither has attempted to measure tone.[4, 18] Each of the reports focused on the ability of the DAFO to alter selected biomechanical variables of walking. Both studies gave a favorable impression of the DAFO when parameters such as total foot contact area or gait velocity were considered, although problems in research design limit the applicability of these results. Although both reports address the use of a DAFO, it is important to note that the design features of each of these orthoses differed.[4, 18]

The DAFO is a flexible brace that allows triplanar movement about the ankle and subtalar joints. Its flexibility is allowed by the $\frac{3}{32}$-inch polypropylene material used in its fabrication. Its supramalleolar height offers the greatest stability for subtalar joint inversion and eversion but does not offer direct control of sagittal plane tibial motion. The walls of the DAFO are trimmed anteriorly and posteriorly to allow for motion into dorsiflexion and plantarflexion, respectively. The customized foot plate of the DAFO is fabricated to maintain a neutral alignment of the ankle and subtalar joints and to offer total contact support to the natural arches of the foot through build-ups in these areas. A small build-up is also made under the toes to facilitate metatarsal alignment, to decrease toe-clawing tendencies, and to enhance an improved dynamic balance response in single-limb support. The total contact design of the brace provides continuous proprioceptive feedback to the user.

DYNAMIC ANKLE ORTHOSIS. The dynamic ankle orthosis or medial ankle support is an orthotic design capable of providing mediolateral stability about the hindfoot in both swing and stance[17, 27] (Fig. 8–14). It is used primarily to reduce subtalar joint inversion and to reestablish a proper base of support from weight acceptance through single-limb support. This design, which consists of a foot plate, short medial upright, and cuff, is made of a single piece of Polyflex II (Smith & Nephew Roylan, Menomonee Falls, WI), which is a flexible plastic material. All measurements and tracings taken prior to fabrication are done with the patient sitting with the feet flat on the floor and the ankles in approximately 10 degrees of dorsiflexion. The subtalar joint is held in neutral alignment.

The medial wall of the dynamic foot orthosis is contoured to grasp the calcaneus to facilitate the desired eversion response during weight acceptance. Shock absorption and forward tibial progression are encouraged over a more stable base of support. As the user progresses into single-limb support, the design of the brace prevents the calcaneus from moving into excessive varus. Single-limb stability is therefore improved, as is hindfoot alignment. This improvement indirectly affects other lower-extremity joint alignments and facilitates normal tibial advancement.

In addition to the stance phase control offered by this orthosis, swing phase ankle and subtalar joint positioning can also be affected. The support offered by the dynamic foot orthosis in swing is adequate to align the ankle

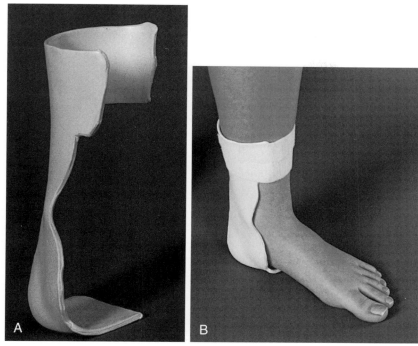

FIGURE 8–14. *A*, The flexible dynamic ankle orthosis consists of a foot plate for calcaneal alignment, a medial upright, and a calf band. *B*, A patient wearing the dynamic ankle orthosis.

in a neutral position with slight eversion at the subtalar joint, even in the presence of mild equinovarus posturing. This positioning assists with foot clearance in midswing and aligns the heel for weight acceptance as previously described.

This type of brace does not limit or directly control the rate or excursion of ankle motion. Potential wearers must have adequate control of tibial advancement and adequate hip and knee stability in stance. The flexibility offered by the dynamic ankle orthosis provides a considerable advantage over more rigid designs because it does not impose any mobility restrictions to daily functional activities. The flexibility of the dynamic ankle orthosis also allows the wearer to use an ankle strategy when needed for balance.

TOE SPREADER. The toe spreader is an orthotic insert consisting of a compressible closed-cell foam plantar insert that is covered with moleskin[17, 26, 27] (Fig. 8–15). It is held in place by four strips of moleskin that are pulled between each of the toes and secured to an additional piece of moleskin that lies on the dorsum of the foot. The placement of the toe spreader along the plantar surface of the foot assists in realigning the toes during single-limb support so that adequate extension and abduction can be attained.

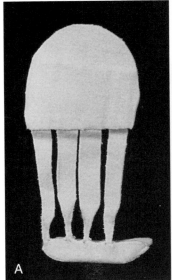
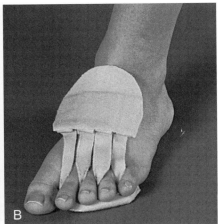

FIGURE 8–15. *A*, The toe spreader consists of a plantar insert made of compressible foam that is covered in moleskin. *B*, Improved toe alignment is achieved by the design of the insert and the interdigital moleskin strips that are pulled to the foot dorsum.

The primary goal of this insert is to reduce toe clawing. By design, it is also effective in reducing the tendency of the forefoot to assume a varus attitude. For the insert to be effective in managing both of these problems, which are frequently encountered together, both must be flexible deformities. Correction of one or both of these flexible deformities reestablishes the base of support across the entire foot in midstance, contributing to overall limb stability. The ability to progress onto the forefoot in terminal stance is enhanced as a result of the realignment offered by the toe spreader. These improvements in the base of support of the foot indirectly promote tibial advancement during both mid- and terminal stance. The toe spreader can be worn by itself or can be used within other orthotic designs when toe realignment is a goal.

KNEE-ANKLE-FOOT ORTHOSES: INDICATIONS, DESIGN, AND COMPONENTS

Generalizations about the population of patients with neurologic involvement are difficult to make because the spectrum of impairments and resultant disabilities tends to be wide across all diagnoses. With respect to orthotic management, however, most adult patients with neurologic involvement require bracing at the below-knee level to manage their walking deficits.

Patients who have a spinal cord injury, polio, or a progressive neurologic condition may require the use of a knee-ankle-foot orthosis (KAFO) if adequate stabilization of the lower extremity cannot be accomplished with a distal design. Because the energy cost of walking with such equipment is great,[20] bracing above the knee is a decision that the rehabilitation team should take seriously. On the other hand, the psychologic benefits of such a decision are certainly important to consider. The discussion that follows highlights some of the major KAFO bracing concepts and components.

Indications for KAFO Prescription

The primary indication for prescribing a KAFO in the population of neurologically impaired adults is the severe and persistent inability to stabilize the knee at weight acceptance and through the single-limb support subphases. The single most common motor control deficit contributing to this problem is that of quadriceps weakness grading fair+ or less on manual muscle examination.[20] Because the hip extensors and ankle plantarflexors are also capable of controlling the sagittal plane relationship of the femur to the tibia throughout the gait cycle, weaknesses of these muscle groups may also contribute to knee instability. This instability may result in excessive knee flexion and buckling, frequent falls, overuse pain, or even progressive weakness. When possible, a patient may actively compensate for this knee instability by avoiding knee flexion in loading response and by thrusting the tibia posteriorly into an extended posture. This movement involves ankle plantarflexion, knee extension or hyperextension, and thigh extension and results in a reduction in the hip flexion angle at loading. The clinical manifestation of the persistent use of this extension thrust strategy over time in the presence of weakness is strain on the posterior knee ligaments.[21] Because of the abnormal loading, these ligaments eventually fail in their intended function, leading to hyperextension range of motion at the knee. A KAFO is indicated in this situation to provide knee stability, to prevent excessive ligamentous strain, and to minimize the joint pain that frequently accompanies this clinical scenario.

Another indication for the use of a KAFO is in the case of impaired or absent proprioception at the knee. This impairment results in knee instability unless the patient actively compensates for it. Likely compensations involve either visually attending to the position of the knee in space or using an extension thrust strategy with weight acceptance to ensure a stable knee alignment.

The reader is referred to the section addressing the challenges of upright function for the neurologically involved adult for a more detailed discussion of the ramifications of stance phase excessive knee flexion and genu recurvatum and their effect on swing limb advancement.

Energy Cost Considerations

The energy cost of ambulation with one or two KAFOs has been well documented as it pertains to the patient with paraplegia caused by a spinal cord injury.[31] Patients with complete injuries walking with bilateral KAFOs and a swing-through crutch-assisted gait pattern demonstrate close to a 500% greater oxygen cost per meter walked, measured in ml/kg/meter, than normal subjects. Gait velocity is 29 meters/minute, compared with the normal walking velocity of 80 meters/minute. The reduced walking efficiency and speed do not meet the functional requirements of normal community ambulation, which entails negotiating distances on average that are greater than 300 meters and gait velocities approaching 80 meters/minute.[13] It is not surprising that many patients with paraplegia choose wheelchair mobility over ambulation as a more efficient mode of transport.

The KAFO is rarely a viable option for the patient with motor control deficits as a result of a cerebrovascular accident or a traumatic brain injury. Even in the presence of knee instability, these patients can be successfully managed with an AFO and appropriate gait-training strategies. This allows the patient to retain a higher degree of function without being encumbered by the proximal uprights of the brace, the additional weight, and the difficulties associated with controlling swing limb advancement. On occasion, a patient with traumatic brain injury with concomitant ligamentous damage to the knee may require the additional stabilization offered by the KAFO to prevent excessive joint play in the involved directions.

Design Principles Used in the KAFO

A three-point pressure system is typically used in the design of a KAFO to prevent knee flexion during stance (Fig. 8–16). The three points of control that stabilize the knee include the posterior aspect of the proximal thigh band, the anterior knee, and the posterior portion of the shoe.[3] Ideal alignment of the KAFO is in full knee extension.

A KAFO designed to provide control for genu recurvatum uses the same three-point pressure system, but the key points of control are modified. In this case, pressure is applied through points of contact along the anterior proximal thigh, through the toe area via the shoe, and posterior to the knee[3] (Fig. 8–17). To promote a stable alignment in stance, the KAFO is aligned in slight recurvatum.

KAFO Components

Both metal and plastic components can be used in the fabrication of a KAFO. The distal components that have been described for the BiCAAL AFO can easily be incorporated into a metal KAFO design. The adjustability offered by this ankle joint is advantageous in the design of a KAFO because

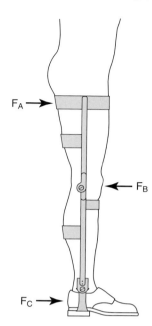

FIGURE 8-16. The design of a knee-ankle-foot orthosis (KAFO) uses a three-point pressure system to control excessive knee flexion in stance. The arrows depict the three lines of force (F_A, F_B, and F_C) required for knee stability.

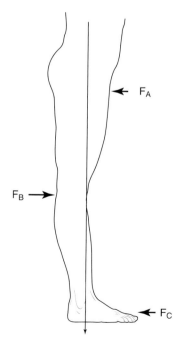

FIGURE 8-17. Three-point pressure system concept applied to the design of a knee-ankle-foot orthosis (KAFO) for the prevention of genu recurvatum.

it allows flexibility with weight acceptance and tibial control during single-limb support. To reduce the overall weight of the KAFO, the distal component may consist of solid plastic. Shoe modifications become especially important in a solid plastic design to facilitate the transition from initial contact to loading response because the adjustability options offered by the metal joint are no longer available.

A number of knee joint options are available to meet the alignment and functional needs of the patient. For example, if the brace has been prescribed to prevent or to minimize genu recurvatum, knee flexion does not need to be limited during gait. A free-motion knee joint provides unlimited knee flexion and prevents genu recurvatum, in addition to providing medio-lateral knee stability[6, 16] (Fig. 8–18A). An offset knee joint can also be used to prevent excessive genu recurvatum while still allowing free knee flexion for functional activities (Fig. 8–18B). The advantage of the offset knee joint is that the mechanical axis of the brace is placed posterior to the anatomic knee joint. The moment arm of the ground-reaction force vector is therefore

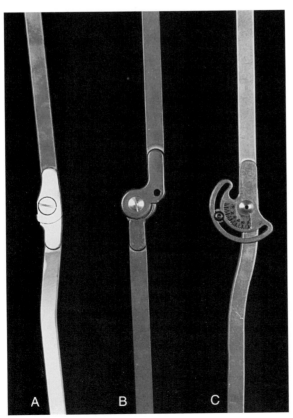

FIGURE 8–18. Examples of knee joints used in knee-ankle-foot orthosis (KAFO) design: *A*, A free-motion knee joint; *B*, the offset knee joint; *C*, the adjustable knee joint.

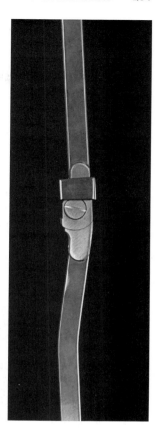

FIGURE 8–19. The ring or drop lock consists of a free-motion knee joint with a ring that can be slid into place over it to prevent knee flexion.

increased in single-limb support. This increases the extension moment at the knee and reduces the need to align the KAFO in excessive hyperextension to achieve stability.[3]

The patient who tends to collapse into excessive limb flexion in stance will require a different knee joint mechanism that can be locked into extension. The most common knee joint used to restrain excessive knee flexion is the ring or drop lock.[6, 16] This joint consists of a basic free-motion knee joint with a metal ring on both the medial and lateral uprights that drops into place to lock the knee once it is extended (Fig. 8–19). The patient can lock the joint for stability in gait but then must unlock it to flex the knees to resume sitting. This movement requires coordinated upper-extremity function.

Another type of knee locking mechanism is the bail or pawl lock, which consists of a semicircular lever that extends posteriorly from the knee joint[6, 16] (Fig. 8–20). When this lever is pulled up, the lock is released and the knee is free to flex. This lock requires less upper-extremity skill to operate. The lock can also be released when upward pressure from the sitting surface is

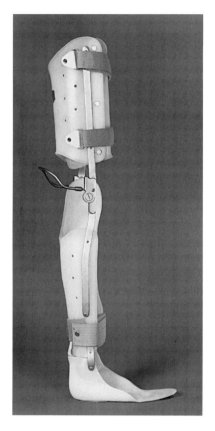

FIGURE 8-20. The bail or pawl knee lock.

applied to the bail. Drawbacks to this design are that the bail lock can be released inadvertently and the device is not cosmetically appealing to some users.

There are also adjustable knee joint designs to accommodate the unique needs of the user. This type of design allows individual adjustment options to limit both flexion and extension range of knee motion. This option can be especially useful when a patient's impairments and function are changing (Fig. 8–18*C*).

Both the height and depth of the bands affect the alignment stability of the KAFO. The proximal thigh band should extend approximately $\frac{1}{2}$ to 1 inch below the ischial tuberosity when the patient is standing. This height is critical to ensure a stable, extended alignment in weight bearing. The band should be well contoured and should fit snugly to the patient's leg. The distal thigh band and the calf band offer control in preventing genu recurvatum. An anterior prepatellar band molded of plastic and fastened with Velcro provides additional control of tibial motion.[21]

ASSESSMENT OF FIT AND FUNCTION

Regardless of the type of bracing that might be prescribed, its effectiveness and overall fit must be assessed frequently. The evaluation should be done with the patient in a static standing position as well as while performing various functional tasks under certain conditions. The primary focus of the static evaluation entails an assessment of orthotic alignment, the fit of any circumferential leg bands such as a calf or thigh cuff, overall patient comfort, and any skin areas that may be experiencing excessive pressures. These same assessments should be made as the patient begins to ambulate because problems may develop only in a dynamic situation.

Observation while the patient is walking provides immediate feedback regarding the effectiveness of the orthosis in remediating gait deviations. The patient should be observed for the emergence of any new gait deviations that might result from the alignment or range-of-motion limitations imposed by the brace. The gait assessment provides critical input that should direct the focus of the patient's ambulation training both with and without the use of the orthosis. Observational gait analysis also directs clinical decisions regarding the need for any footwear modifications or orthotic adjustments related to alignment or movement availability.

As was previously discussed in this chapter, the gait subphase of loading response poses a significant challenge to the ambulatory subject. These challenges may be magnified for the orthotic wearer in certain situations. For example, a rigid brace design that prevents ankle movement does not allow a normal plantarflexion response following heel contact. As a result, tibial forward progression will be quick and abrupt, forcing the knee and subsequently the hip into a flexed posture that is likely to be excessive.[12] If the patient is wearing a DAAJ AFO that is locked, the addition of a cushioned heel may assist in reducing this knee flexion thrust at loading. This type of heel tends to wear out quickly, however. A beveled heel is another shoe modification that reduces the impact of loading body weight onto a rigid ankle. By beveling or undercutting the heel, the clinician can reduce the lever arm of the heel, thereby reducing the knee flexion moment at loading[15] (Fig. 8–21). This same effect can be achieved by using a running shoe that has a beveled heel in its design.

Orthotic evaluation should also include assessment of the patient's gait at varying speeds and across a range of terrain options. Gait deviations that appear to have only a minimal effect on walking at the patient's comfortable walking speed may be grossly exaggerated as speed increases. An extensor thrust, which involves a forceful extension of the knee, is a common clinical example of a gait deviation that is frequently exacerbated by an increased gait velocity. Again, shoe modifications or brace alignment adjustments may be required to meet these changing needs. Similarly, the impact of the orthosis should be considered as it affects activities requiring a range of ankle movements, such as stair climbing, sidestepping, or walking backward.

A

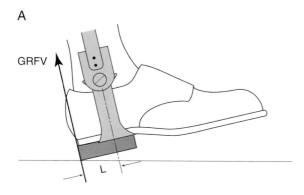

B

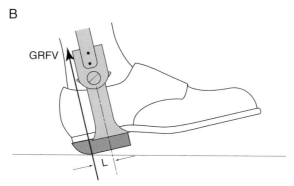

FIGURE 8–21. *A*, The heel lever (L) in a shoe with a standard heel. This lever represents the perpendicular distance from the axis of the orthotic ankle joint to the ground-reaction force vector (GRFV). *B*, Beveling the heel reduces its lever and smoothes the transition into a flat foot position by reducing the resultant knee flexion moment.

The patient may need to make some adjustments in movement patterns to perform these activities with an orthosis. The goal of functional training should be to assist the patient in efficiently handling these situations.

Single- and double-limb support balance needs to be assessed, especially if ankle joint movement is restricted by the orthosis. Limitations in ankle range of motion may affect the patient's ability to effectively recruit an ankle strategy when balance is challenged. An orthosis wearer may therefore be forced into using a hip strategy to recover from a perturbation that might otherwise be handled primarily at the ankle joint.

Progression of Brace Design and Adjustment

The ever-changing clinical picture of the adult neurologic patient requires an equally progressive response in determining the patient's bracing requirements. An ongoing assessment of the patient's function across a range of activities provides an objective means of analyzing the appropriateness of the current bracing design and its potential shortcomings as further neurologic recovery is attained. Minor brace adjustments or footwear modifications may be necessary to optimize the patient's current brace design.

The goal of orthotic intervention is based on the individual needs of the patient and the environment in which he or she will be functioning. In the early management of an adult with neurologic involvement, the orthotic goal may center around the ability to optimize weight bearing in the foot so that sitting and standing activities can be emphasized. This foot position facilitates the patient's ability to move over the base of support as proximal control is emphasized. The ambulatory patient who has severe physical deficits may benefit from the use of an orthosis that provides maximal distal stabilization so that trunk and hip control can be emphasized during dynamic gait activities. The brace may also provide safety to the patient and the joint structure by means of stabilizing the foot in stance and preventing injury that could result from an abnormal weight-bearing posture. Orthotic use can be especially helpful when dealing with the patient who has severe bilateral involvement. Orthoses may provide improved lower-extremity alignment while allowing the joint mobility required for function.

As the adult patient progresses in the recovery process, therapeutic goals frequently focus on the ability to make transitional movements smoothly and to function in an upright posture. In this case, a brace may be viewed as a tool that helps to prevent abnormal alignments, yet encourages maximal mobility whenever possible. As further progress is made, the role of the orthosis may simply be to provide minimal alignment assistance or stabilization during dynamic activities.

SUMMARY

Current trends in movement analysis and reeducation have begun to draw our attention away from addressing treatment goals that focus on changing isolated symptoms of movement dysfunction, such as muscle tone, reflex activity, or single joint problems.[7] Rather, greater emphasis is being placed on analyzing and treating the essential components of functional movement, which include the base of support, alignment, sequencing, and issues of stability and mobility. An orthosis may alter any or all of these biomechanical considerations related to movement. Kinematic and kinetic analyses provide us with an opportunity to confirm the efficacy of orthotic intervention related to these movement components. Further research is needed to document and to describe the kinematic and kinetic changes that occur during functional transitions and walking when an orthosis is applied to an adult with neurologic involvement.

Orthotic prescription involves matching an individual's functional requirements to a bracing design that enables optimal responsiveness. Choices must be made regarding the type of materials involved in the design of the orthosis, its overall alignment, and its ability to be modified or adjusted. Footwear choices are equally important because they directly influence the ability of the brace to provide stability or to allow mobility of a specific body segment. Successful orthotic management involves ongoing assessment and progression over time to address the changing functional requirements of the individual with neurologic involvement.

REFERENCES

1. Bohannon RW: Gait performance of hemiparetic stroke patients: Selected variables. Arch Phys Med Rehabil 68:777–781, 1987.
2. Cerny K: Pathomechanics of stance. Clinical concepts for analysis. Phys Ther 64:1851–1859, 1984.
3. Clark D: Knee ankle foot orthosis design for polio. In Rancho Los Amigos Medical Center Prosthetics and Orthotics Course Syllabus: Critical Decisions in Patient Management. Downey, CA, Professional Staff Association, 6:60–62, 1985.
4. Diamond MF, Ottenbacher KJ: Effect of a tone-inhibiting dynamic ankle-foot orthosis on stride characteristics of an adult with hemiparesis. Phys Ther 70:423–430, 1990.
5. Duer R: Orthotic management of moderate equinovarus. In Rancho Los Amigos Medical Center Prosthetics and Orthotics Course Syllabus: Critical Decisions in Patient Management. Downey, CA, Professional Staff Association, 6:19–24, 1985.
6. Edelstein JE: Orthotic assessment and management. In O'Sullivan SB, Schmitz TJ (eds): Physical Rehabilitation: Assessment and Treatment, Philadelphia, F.A. Davis Co., 1988, pp 589–614.
7. Fisher B, Yakura J: Movement analysis. A different perspective. Orthop Phys Ther Clin North Am 2:1–14, 1993.
8. Hylton NM: Postural and functional impact of dynamic AFOs and FOs in a pediatric population. J Prosthet Orthot 2(1):40–53, 1989.
9. Kloos AD: Measurement of muscle tone and strength. Neurol Rep 1:9–12, 1992.
10. Lehmann JF: Push-off and propulsion of the body in normal and abnormal gait. Correction by ankle-foot orthoses. Clin Orthop 288:97–108, 1993.
11. Lehmann JF, Condon SM, Price R, et al: Gait abnormalities in hemiplegia: Their correction by ankle-foot orthoses. Arch Phys Med Rehabil 68:763–771, 1987.
12. Lehmann JF, Esselman PC, Ko MJ, et al: Plastic ankle-foot orthoses: Evaluation of function. Arch Phys Med Rehabil 64:402–407, 1983.
13. Lerner-Frankiel MB, Vargas S, Brown M, et al: Functional community ambulation: What are your criteria? Clin Management 6(2):12–15, 1986.
14. Lohman M, Goldstein H: Alternative strategies in tone-reducing AFO design. J Prosthet Orthot 5(1):1–4, 1993.
15. Lunsford BR, Gentile C: Gait penalties of inadequate calf control: Spinal cord injury (vigorous walker). In Rancho Los Amigos Medical Center Prosthetics and Orthotics Course Syllabus: Critical Decisions in Patient Management. Downey, CA, Professional Staff Association, 6:42–49, 1985.
16. Lunsford T: Orthotic principles. In Rancho Los Amigos Medical Center Prosthetics and Orthotics Course Syllabus: Critical Decisions in Patient Management. Downey, CA, Professional Staff Association, 6:1–9, 1985.
17. Montgomery J: Orthotic management of the lower limb in head-injured adults. J Head Trauma Rehabil 2:57–61, 1987.
18. Mueller K, Cornwall M, McPoil T, et al: Effect of a tone-inhibiting dynamic ankle-foot orthosis on the foot-loading pattern of a hemiplegic adult: A preliminary study. J Prosthet Orthot 4(2):86–92, 1992.
19. Pathokinesiology Service, Physical Therapy Department: Observational Gait Analysis, Downey, CA, Los Amigos Research and Education Institute, Inc, 1993.

20. Perry J: Gait Analysis: Normal and Pathological Function, New York, McGraw-Hill Book Co., 1992.
21. Perry J: Knee ankle foot orthoses. Clinical illustration: Polio. In Rancho Los Amigos Medical Center Prosthetics and Orthotics Course Syllabus: Critical Decisions in Patient Management. Downey, CA, Professional Staff Association, 6:57–59, 1985.
22. Schenkman M, Berger RA, Riley PO, et al: Whole-body movements during rising to standing from sitting. Phys Ther 70:638–651, 1990.
23. Shamp JK: Neurophysiologic orthotic designs in the treatment of central nervous system disorders. J Prosthet Orthot 2(1):14–32, 1989.
24. Shumway-Cook A, Woollacott M (eds): Motor Control. Theory and Practical Applications, Baltimore, Williams & Wilkins, 1995.
25. Skinner SR, Antonelli D, Perry J, et al: Functional demands on the stance limb in walking. Orthopedics 8(3):355–361, 1985.
26. Utley J, Thomas CS: Orthotic management of the lower extremity. In Montgomery J (ed): Physical Therapy for Traumatic Brain Injury, New York, Churchill Livingstone, Inc, 1995, pp 137–160.
27. Utley J, Woll S: Orthotics Used with the NDT (Bobath) Approach to Neurologic Patients. Course Syllabus. Chicago, Rehabilitation Institute of Chicago, 1995.
28. Waters RL: Passive dropfoot clinical illustration: Trauma. In Rancho Los Amigos Medical Center Prosthetics and Orthotics Course Syllabus: Critical Decisions in Patient Management. Downey, CA, Professional Staff Association, 6:10–12, 1985.
29. Waters RL, Garland DE, Montgomery J: Orthotic prescription for stroke and head injury. In American Academy of Orthopedic Surgeons: Atlas of Orthotics. Biomechanical Principles and Application, St. Louis, CV Mosby, 1985, pp 270–286.
30. Waters RL, Lunsford BR: Energy expenditure of normal and pathologic gait: Application to orthotic prescription. In American Academy of Orthopedic Surgeons: Atlas of Orthotics. Biomechanical Principles and Application, St. Louis, CV Mosby, 1985, pp 151–159.
31. Waters RL, Yakura JS: The energy expenditure of normal and pathologic gait. Crit Rev Phys Rehabil Med 1(3):183–209, 1989.
32. Zachazewski JE, Eberle ED, Jefferies M: Effect of tone-inhibiting casts and orthoses on gait. A case report. Phys Ther 62:453–455, 1982.

CHAPTER 9

Use of Orthoses
in Pediatrics

MEG STANGER

The use of orthoses in the pediatric population must take several factors into consideration, in particular the fact that a child's musculoskeletal system, in contrast to that of an adult's, is growing and developing. The growth and development of the musculoskeletal system occur through a balanced interplay between the physiologic properties of bone and soft tissue and biomechanical forces, and any alterations in this balance may result in secondary deformities or functional limitations.[8, 22] A knowledge of growth and development of the musculoskeletal system and the influence of physiologic and biomechanical forces on that system is therefore essential to understand the purpose, influence, and efficacy of orthoses with children.

This chapter will briefly discuss the normal growth and development of bone and soft tissues, the use of orthoses to promote treatment goals and improve function, and the limitations of orthotics for the pediatric population.

MUSCULOSKELETAL DEVELOPMENT

The prenatal formation and development of the musculoskeletal system is well documented in the literature and is beyond the scope of this chapter. However, the clinician treating the pediatric population needs to have a thorough knowledge of the prenatal and postnatal growth and development of the musculoskeletal system in order to determine appropriate intervention strategies. Orthotic devices may have beneficial or detrimental effects on growing children, depending on the goals for the orthosis, the timing of the intervention, and the duration of the intervention.

The shape of the skeleton is determined by the cartilaginous model laid down during the fetal period. During the second month of gestation, the cartilaginous skeleton begins to be replaced by bone through the process of endochondral ossification. Movement, either prenatally or postnatally, generates mechanical forces that affect the size and shape of bones. These forces act on the fetal skeleton and continue to act on the immature musculoskeletal system of the growing child.

Compressive forces act perpendicularly to the epiphyseal plate and stimulate longitudinal growth. Examples of normal compressive forces include weight bearing and muscle pulls associated with contractions or movement. If compressive forces become too great, longitudinal bone growth may be retarded. Asymmetric bone growth may be the result of forces acting unequally across the epiphyseal plate; compressive forces may be increased in one area and retard growth, whereas the same forces may be decreased in another area and stimulate growth. The bone may appear to be bending but is actually growing asymmetrically.[1, 37] Valgus and varus deformities may be the result of unequal forces or loading across the epiphyseal plate.

Compressive forces also affect the size and density of bones because they stimulate appositional growth. An increase in weight bearing increases the density of the shaft of the bone, whereas a decrease in or lack of weight bearing leads to a reduction in bone density and increases the risk of osteoporosis.[1]

Shearing forces act parallel to the epiphyseal plate, causing newly formed bone to grow away from the epiphysis in a spiral pattern, producing a torsion of the bone.[37] The normal pull of muscles around a joint will affect torsional changes seen during growth and development of infants and young children. Infants are born with 5 degrees of medial tibial rotation. Normal muscle pull on a developing and growing tibia produces approximately 23 to 25 degrees of lateral tibial rotation by adulthood.[8]

Compressive and shear forces normally act on the immature musculoskeletal system to change the shapes and angles of bones. These changes lead to the mature model of the skeleton and the efficient biomechanical functioning of the adult skeleton. The musculoskeletal system is, however, driven by the nervous system, and with neurologic damage, alterations in the direction and strength of muscle pull and weight bearing can occur. These alterations will apply abnormal forces on the immature musculoskeletal system and may produce deformities such as vertebral wedging, hip subluxations or dislocations, femoral anteversion, tibial torsion, genu varus or valgus, and rearfoot and midfoot alignment problems. Deformities of the musculoskeletal system can lead to impairments, functional limitations, and eventually disability.

Several factors will assist in the determination of an appropriate orthosis for a child. The goals of the treatment and limitations of the orthotic device must be clearly understood. The goals for children are similar to those for adults and may include (1) maintenance of joint range of motion or prevention of contracture, (2) correction of deformity, (3) protection or stabilization of a joint, (4) promotion of joint alignment, (5) restoration of function, and (6) promotion of function. The child's age and the stage of development of the musculoskeletal system will also have an impact on the orthotic decision.

USE OF ORTHOSES FOR CONGENITAL OR ACQUIRED ABNORMALITIES OF BONE

Congenital Hip Dysplasia (Developmental Hip Dysplasia)

Several mechanical and physiologic conditions predispose neonates to congenital hip dysplasia (CHD). Many of the factors are related to in utero space restrictions in the last trimester of the pregnancy or to a restriction of fetal movement. These conditions, which cause the fetus to be wedged in the maternal pelvis with the hip in a flexed and adducted posture,[26] include tight maternal abdominal and intrauterine musculature (in the case of firstborns), breech presentation, and decreased amniotic fluid, all of which are associated with an increased incidence of CHD.

At the time of birth, the hip joint is the most unstable joint in the body. The acetabulum is shallow and covers less than one half of the femoral head. In addition, the joint capsule is distended and elastic, allowing the femoral head to sublux from under the shallow acetabulum. After birth, the depth of the acetabulum increases, and the femoral head becomes more spheric, creating a more stable joint. Kicking movements pre- and postnatally are theorized to assist with the development and shaping of both the acetabulum and the femoral head.[63]

When a hip subluxation or dislocation is recognized in the newborn, the femoral head can be relocated readily, and the shape of the joint and soft tissues will be nearly normal. However, if the hip is left untreated, secondary joint and soft tissue deformities will develop. The longer the hip is left untreated, the greater will be the severity of the deformities. The femoral head migrates proximally and laterally along the pelvis because of the normal pull of the hip flexor and hip adductor muscle groups. The acetabulum becomes flatter without the stimulation of the femoral head to increase the depth. Muscle contractures may develop with the hip adductor, hip flexor, and hamstring muscle groups. Eventually, the femoral head may become misshapen and flatter as it rubs against the pelvis. The contact of the femoral head will produce a false acetabulum along the lateral wall of the pelvis.[26]

The goal of treatment in CHD is to return the femoral head to its normal position in the acetabulum and maintain this position until the pathologic changes are reversed. The femoral head must first be relocated in the acetabulum and then maintained in a position of hip flexion and abduction.[26] Several orthotic devices have been developed to maintain the hip reduction, and most of these can achieve successful results if they are applied properly. However, if applied incorrectly, the orthoses may produce complications such as redislocation or avascular necrosis. Forced or excessive hip abduction may occlude the medial circumflex artery, resulting in avascular necrosis of the femoral head.[63]

Pavlik Harness

The Pavlik harness consists of a shoulder harness, stirrups for the legs, and booties to hold the feet (Fig. 9–1). The device is fabricated from a washable canvas material and secured with Velcro straps. Buckles on the straps allow for growth of the infant. The anterior strap on the leg allows hip flexion but limits hip extension. The posterior leg strap limits hip adduction and allows hip abduction. The Pavlik harness is a dynamic splint that allows active hip motions of flexion and abduction to locate the femoral head and shape the acetabulum.[48, 60] The incidence of avascular necrosis with use of the Pavlik harness has been reported by several authors as negligible or nonexistent if

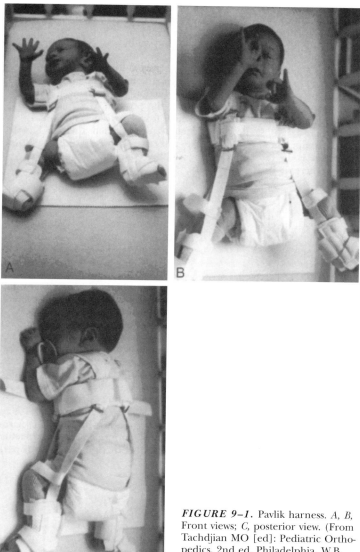

FIGURE 9–1. Pavlik harness. *A, B,* Front views; *C,* posterior view. (From Tachdjian MO [ed]: Pediatric Orthopedics, 2nd ed, Philadelphia, W.B. Saunders Co., 1990.)

it is used for the correct indications and if the application instructions are followed.[32, 48, 60]

Frejka Pillow

The Frejka pillow is a bulky device, resembling a triple set of diapers, that is placed between the legs of the child (Fig. 9–2). The pillow must be reapplied

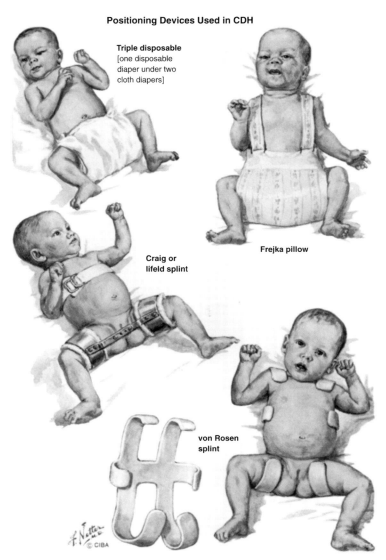

FIGURE 9–2. Orthoses for management of congenital hip dysplasia. (From Hensinger RN: Congenital dislocation of the hip. CIBA Clin Symp 31:15, 1979. ©Copyright 1996. CIBA-GEIGY Corporation. Reprinted with permission from the Clinical Symposia illustrated by Frank Netter, M.D. All rights reserved.)

after each diaper change. With frequent changes of the pillow, the femoral head may sublux or dislocate and go unnoticed by the caregiver. The Frejka pillow also increases the risk of excessive abduction and the development of avascular necrosis.[60]

Craig or Ilfeld Splint

The Craig or Ilfeld splint maintains the hips in flexion and abduction and does not need to be removed with each diaper change (see Fig. 9–2). This splint is secured only around the infant's thighs and does not have a component securing it over the infant's shoulders. It therefore tends to slip distally. This slippage necessitates constant readjustment and may threaten the location of the femoral head.[60]

von Rosen Splint

The von Rosen splint is fabricated of soft metal and is covered by soft padding (see Fig. 9–2). The splint surrounds the thighs, holding the hips in flexion and abduction. Shoulder extensions prevent the splint from sliding on the legs. The flexible metal allows the splint to be fitted individually and also permits some hip mobility. If the splint is fitted loosely, the infant may kick in flexion and abduction; the splint serves only to block hip adduction and extension movements.[60] The advantages of the von Rosen splint over the previously mentioned orthoses are that the shoulder extensions on the splint prohibit the sliding of the splint down the legs, and that fitting the splints loosely allows the infant to kick actively, thereby possibly assisting with the shaping of the femoral head and acetabulum.

A complication of the von Rosen splint is the development of facial nerve paralysis. Tachdjian[60] reported that young infants with limited head control may tilt the head against the metal stirrups at the shoulders, causing pressure to build over the mastoid process. However, this problem appears to be eliminated if the metal stirrups are well padded. The incidence of avascular necrosis with the von Rosen splint is significantly lower than with the Frejka pillow.[25]

Legg-Calvé-Perthes Disease

Legg-Calvé-Perthes disease is a self-limiting disease of the hip initiated by avascular necrosis of the femoral head. The disease occurs in children between 3 and 13 years of age, with a male-to-female ratio of 4:1. Legg-Calvé-Perthes disease is most commonly seen in boys between 5 and 7 years of age.[13, 15] The cause of this disease is not known, but several factors such as trauma, infection, and transient synovitis have been linked to avascular necrosis.[13]

Legg-Calvé-Perthes disease progresses through several stages including the initial stage of avascular necrosis of the femoral head, the resorption stage, and the reparative stage. The resorption and reparative stages involve the resorption of dead bone, revascularization, reossification of the femoral head, and remodeling of the femoral head and acetabulum. This disease process may last between 1 and 3 years. Prognosis for a good outcome is dependent on the age of onset, extent of femoral head involvement, extent of involvement of the physis, and congruency between the femoral head and the acetabulum.[13, 15, 60]

Orthoses for Legg-Calvé-Perthes disease have been used as a containment method of treatment to maintain the femoral head in the acetabulum during the disease process. The goal of containment is to develop a congruent joint with a spheric femoral head and a normally shaped acetabulum.[60]

Scottish-Rite Orthosis

The child's hips are held in 40 to 45 degrees of abduction by two thigh cuffs connected to a crossbar. The crossbar contains a swivel joint that allows reciprocal movement of the legs. Each thigh cuff is attached to a lateral upright with a hip joint and a pelvic band (Fig. 9–3), and the child is able to ambulate using this orthosis. The Scottish-Rite orthosis has become the most commonly prescribed orthosis in North America for the treatment of Legg-Calvé-Perthes disease.[13, 60]

Studies on the effectiveness of the Scottish-Rite orthosis in containing the femoral head in the acetabulum and allowing remodeling have involved small sample sizes and have looked only at the short-term results. These studies demonstrate effectiveness rates of 75% to 90%, depending on the age of the child and the severity of involvement. These rates are comparable to rates attained with other containment treatment methods.[51, 65] The advantages of the Scottish-Rite orthosis are that it is relatively easy to put on and take off, it provides improved mobility (including ambulation) without assistive devices, and it is a less cumbersome, more cosmetically appealing orthosis. Its disadvantage lies in its inability to control hip rotation motions, thereby making it a less appropriate orthosis for children with more severe disease.

Petrie Cast

The Petrie cast is an abduction plaster cast with two wooden abduction bars (Fig. 9–4). Technically, the child may ambulate with crutches while wearing the cast, but ambulation is very difficult and awkward because of the weight of the cast, the widely abducted position of the hips, and the lack of motion at the child's hips and knees. In an initial study of 60 patients by Petrie and Bitnec,[49] the outcome was good in 60%, fair in 31%, and poor in 9% of the patients. The rating scale of good, fair, and poor was developed by Mose and has been discussed by Katz[33] as being an effective and reproducible method of evaluating the shape of the femoral head and coverage of the femoral head by the acetabulum. The results achieved by Petrie can now be obtained with less cumbersome methods of containment such as the Scottish-Rite orthosis.[19]

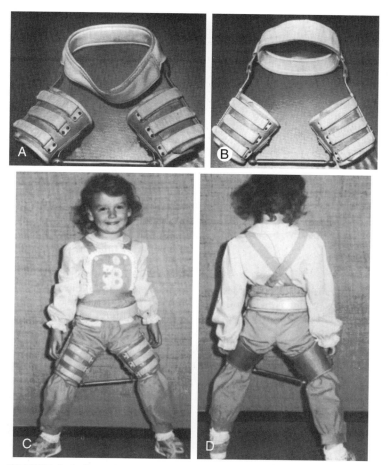

FIGURE 9–3. Scottish-Rite orthosis. *A, B,* Front and posterior views; *C, D,* front and posterior views of a child wearing the orthosis. (From Tachdjian MO [ed]: Pediatric Orthopedics, 2nd ed, Philadelphia, W.B. Saunders Co., 1990.)

Newington Orthosis

The Newington orthosis stabilizes the hips in 45 degrees of abduction and 20 degrees of internal rotation by two full-length medial uprights and leather or Velcro thigh and calf straps. A distal abduction bar maintains the hip abduction (Fig. 9–5). The orthosis is lighter than the Petrie cast, but ambulation remains difficult and awkward, secondary to the widely abducted position of the legs and lack of motion at the child's hips and knees. The outcome, as reported by Curtis and associates,[17] was good in 63%, fair in 21%, and poor in 16% of patients using the Newington orthosis. The Newington orthosis was often used in children with more severe involvement and necrosis of the femoral head. The poorer prognosis for complete

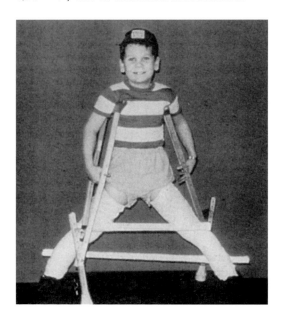

FIGURE 9–4. Petrie cast. (From Canale ST: Osteochondroses. In Canale ST and Beaty JH [eds]: Operative Pediatric Orthopedics, St. Louis, Mosby-Year Book, 1991.)

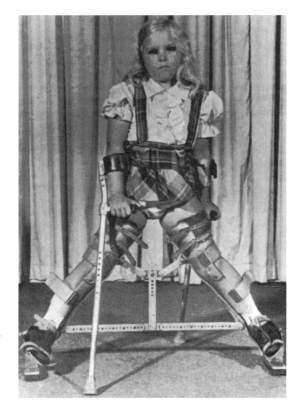

FIGURE 9–5. Newington orthosis. (From Leach RE, Hoaglund FT, Riseborough ET: Controversies in Orthopedic Surgery, Philadelphia, W.B. Saunders Co., 1982.)

healing and remodeling associated with more severe disease may contribute to the lower rate of success with this orthosis compared to rates with other containment orthoses.

Other Treatment

Depending on the severity of disease and their age, many children with Legg-Calvé-Perthes disease do not require treatment. Controversy exists regarding treatments that include the use of orthoses or surgery. Orthoses must be worn for extended periods of up to 2 to 3 years. They are bulky, require the user's compliance over a long period of time, and interfere with the child's normal activity with peers. However, some investigators have reported satisfactory results with remodeling and covering the femoral head in children who wore the orthosis for only 12 to 18 months.[62]

Surgical containment is an option that may be more appealing than an orthosis for some children and their parents. Surgical containment of the head in the acetabulum is a shorter process compared to the 12- to 18-month period that is required with an orthosis to achieve similar results of remodeling of the femoral head and covering of the femoral head by the acetabulum. The risks of surgery must also be considered when comparing orthotic versus surgical techniques. The risks of surgery are specific to the technique performed but may include loss of hip joint range of motion, weakness of the gluteus medius muscle with a subsequent Trendelenburg gait if the procedure is a femoral osteotomy, inequality of leg length secondary to femoral shortening after a femoral osteotomy, and stress fracture below the plate or the screws. Another disadvantage of surgery is the need for a second surgical procedure to remove the hardware after healing has occurred.[60]

Rotational Variations

The normal alignment of the limbs in children is a confusing topic, and one that often causes concern among parents. Parents may raise questions regarding their child's in-toeing or out-toeing and the need for treatment. The causative factors of the in-toeing or out-toeing must be evaluated, and the rotational alignments must be measured to determine whether the values fall within the normal range for the age of the child. An evaluation of in-toeing or out-toeing should include the following: assessment of foot progression angle during gait; measurement of hip rotation or femoral torsion (Ryder's test), thigh-foot angle, and transmalleolar axis; and assessment of foot configuration including subtalar joint alignment and presence of metatarsus adductus.[6, 11, 18, 56, 57] The results of the rotational profile will help determine which components of the lower extremities are contributing to the in-toeing or out-toeing. The normal values for rotational alignment for the age of the child must then be considered (Fig. 9–6). If the rotational values fall within the normal range for a specific age, treatment is not

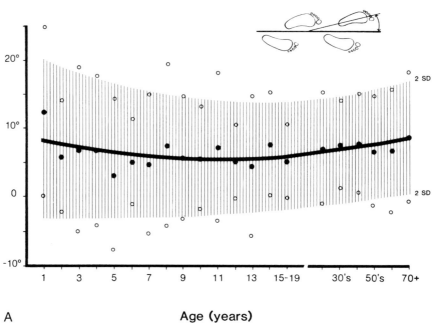

A

Age (years)

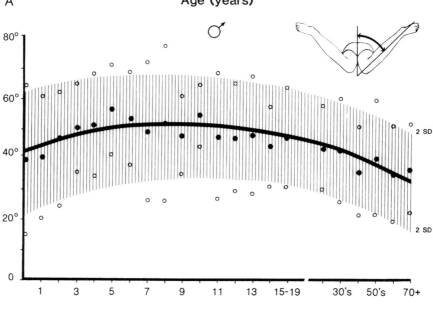

B

Age (years)

FIGURE 9–6. The five measurements plotted as the mean values plus or minus two standard deviations for each of the 22 age groups. The solid lines show the mean changes with age; the shaded areas, the normal ranges; the solid circles, the mean measurements for the different age groups; and the open circles, plus or minus two standard deviations for the same mean measurements. A, Foot-progression angle; B, medial rotation of the hip in male subjects.

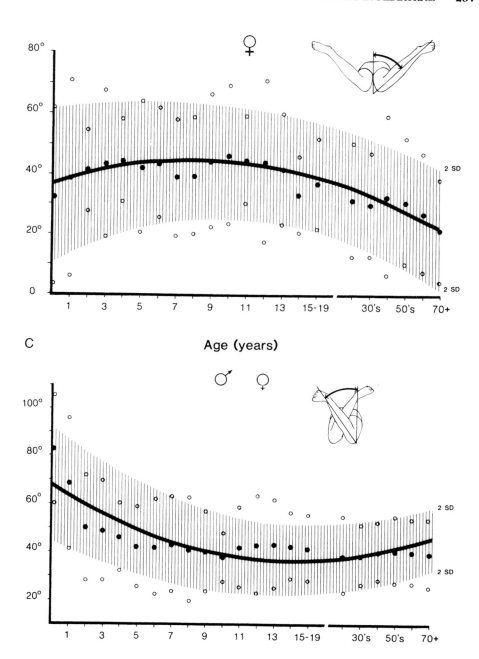

FIGURE 9-6 *Continued C*, Medial rotation of the hip in female subjects; *D*, lateral rotation of the hip in male and female subjects combined.

Illustration continued on following page

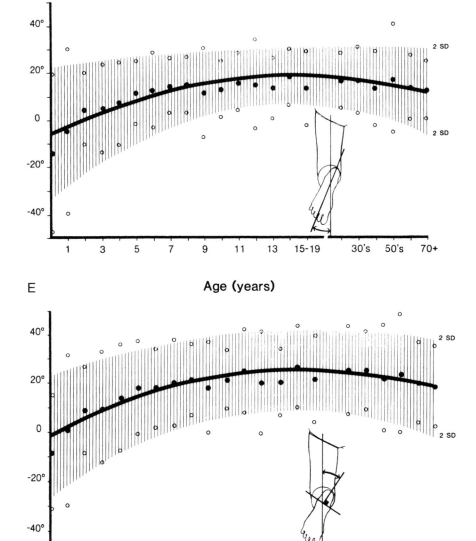

E

Age (years)

F

Age (years)

FIGURE 9–6 *Continued E,* Thigh-foot angle; *F,* angle of the transmalleolar axis. (From Staheli LT, Corbett M, Wyss C, et al: Lower-extremity rotational problems in children. J Bone Joint Surg 67A:39–47, 1985.)

indicated, and the in-toeing or out-toeing will change as the child grows and the musculoskeletal system matures. If the rotational values fall outside the normal rotational variations for a given age by two standard deviations, a torsional deformity does exist and treatment options can be explored.[60] Consideration must also be given to whether the variation from normal values for a specific age will result in functional limitations for the child either at the current time or in the future.

Denis Browne Splint

With the Denis Browne splint the child's shoes are attached to a rigid metal bar (Fig. 9–7). The angle of the attachment of the shoes to the bar is easily adjusted to produce a neutral position or varying degrees of in-toeing or out-toeing. The Denis Browne splint has been used to correct femoral anteversion, tibial torsion, and metatarsus adductus, but its effectiveness in correcting these abnormalities is not documented. Many authors suggest that this orthosis is often unnecessary and produces abnormal stresses on the knee and ankle.[6, 58] A few authors recommend the use of the Denis Browne splint for specific rotational deformities. Tachdjian[60] suggests its use for children with medial tibial torsion that exceeds 40 degrees, with a positive family history of persistent abnormal medial tibial torsion, and with a lack of spontaneous correction with growth.

Shoe Modifications

Orthopedic shoes and lateral sole and heel wedges have been prescribed to correct femoral and tibial rotations. Knittel and Staheli[34] studied 10 children who presented with bilateral in-toeing. Each child was fitted with seven wedge combinations, two Torqheels (Meiller Research Inc., College Station, TX), and a control shoe. The children were videotaped while walking.

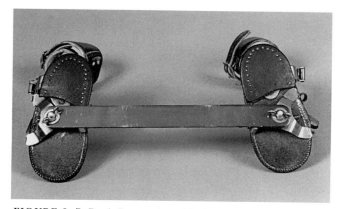

FIGURE 9–7. Denis Browne bar with shoes attached.

Measurements were taken for 100 left and 100 right midstance steps for each child wearing each orthosis and the control shoe. The results showed that none of the shoe modifications significantly altered the angle of in-toeing for the subjects, and the authors concluded that shoe modifications have no clinically significant effect on in-toeing in children.

The literature pertaining to rotational variations remains confusing. Clinicians must assess the child's rotational profile, refer to Staheli's[57] (see Fig. 9–6) graphs of normal values, and determine the method of treatment. Treatment may include no orthotic or surgical intervention because the rotational variation assessed is normal for the child's age and will resolve over the course of normal growth and development. The role of the clinician then is to educate the parents and assure them that treatment would not correct the clinical problem. The use of orthoses for rotational deformities that are two standard deviations outside the normal rotational range cannot be substantiated by the current literature. Surgical techniques such as rotational osteotomies may be indicated for those children who exhibit torsional deformities that will interfere with their ability to function normally in the future.

USE OF FULL LOWER-EXTREMITY ORTHOTIC SYSTEMS

For this discussion, full lower-extremity orthotic systems include standing devices such as parapodiums, hip-knee-ankle-foot orthoses (HKAFOs), and reciprocating gait orthoses (RGOs). These orthotic devices may be used for standing purposes only or for ambulation. See Chapter 2 for further discussion of the RGOs and HKAFOs.

Standing Devices

"Standing devices" is a broad term that includes standing frames, parapodiums, swivel walkers, and supine and prone standers. Each of these devices initially aims to introduce upright positioning to children who cannot stand independently. The goals to be achieved with standing in the pediatric population are similar to those for adults and include improvements in circulation, kidney function, and respiratory status.[12, 20, 55] For the child with an immature musculoskeletal system, standing may also improve bone mass and density and promote normal joint development.

Normal compressive forces that come into play with weight bearing promote the shaping of the acetabulum and the femoral head.[5, 50] The deepening of the acetabulum and the shaping of the femoral head do not occur in nonweight-bearing children with cerebral palsy.[29] Studies have not been conducted on the effect of standing devices on the joint development of children with disabilities.

Standing devices may also be used to promote improved bone density. Nonambulatory children with disabilities often exhibit decreased bone density compared to children without disabilities.[31, 38, 52, 59] In children with myelomeningocele, bone density is greater in those who are ambulatory compared to those who use a wheelchair for mobility.[54] Preliminary studies suggest that the use of a standing device for a 60-minute duration four to five times a week results in increased bone density in nonambulatory children with cerebral palsy.[59]

Studying specific standing devices, Miedaner[44] and Cunningham and associates[16] found that the weight borne by the legs increased as the child came closer to the vertical position. If prone and supine standers are being used with the goal of increasing bone density, these aids need to be used so that the child is inclined within 20 degrees of the vertical position. If the incline is greater than 20 degrees from vertical, the weight tends to be borne through the child's stomach or back. Standing frames, parapodiums, and swivel walkers, unlike the adjustable prone and supine standers, are fabricated so that the child stands vertically within the device (Fig. 9–8).

Parapodiums and swivel walkers may be used as early ambulation devices for children with myelomeningocele.[35] The parapodium resembles a standing frame except that it contains hip and knee locks that accommodate a sitting posture. Using a walker, a child may develop ambulation skills incorporating a swing-through or swing-to gait with a parapodium. Ambulation may also be achieved using a swivel walker and no assistive device.

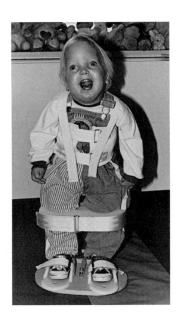

FIGURE 9–8. Standing frame, front view. (From Myers RS [ed]: Saunders Manual of Physical Therapy Practice. Philadelphia, W.B. Saunders Co., 1995.)

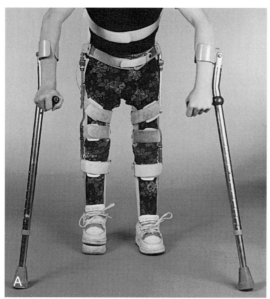

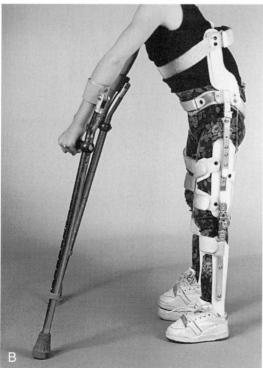

FIGURE 9–9. Hip-knee-ankle-foot orthosis (HKAFO) with thoracic strap. *A*, Front view; *B*, side view.

Forward mobility is accomplished by lateral weight shifts that produce a reciprocal motion of the foot plates. A higher walking velocity can be achieved with the parapodium compared to the swivel walker, but decreased energy cost and a more efficient gait are noted with use of the swivel walker.[39] Gait efficiency was determined from the ratio of the energy cost to the walking velocity. Children using a parapodium for ambulation demonstrated increases or decreases in their velocity when their energy cost increased. Therefore, the energy cost and gait efficiency advantages of the swivel walker may be more important factors for some children compared to the increased walking velocity achieved with the parapodium.

Hip-Knee-Ankle-Foot Orthoses

A description of conventional HKAFOs can be found in Chapter 2. HKAFOs are frequently used with children with myelomeningocele at a motor level involvement of L4 or higher. Children with involvement of motor levels at L1–2 or higher may benefit from extended lateral uprights and the attachment of a thoracic strap (Fig. 9–9). The purpose of the thoracic strap is to limit forward flexion of the trunk and to promote a more upright posture.

Modifications to conventional HKAFOs are necessary if ambulation is to

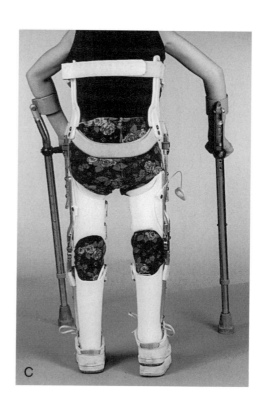

FIGURE 9–9 Continued C, Posterior view.

C

be initiated by a child with moderate to severe osteogenesis imperfecta. The National Institutes of Health Children's Hospital National Medical Center (NIH-CHNMC) program advocates the use of lightweight containment or clamshell orthoses in ambulation for children with moderate to severe osteogenesis imperfecta. Although fractures continue to occur with the containment orthoses, the frequency of fractures is reduced compared to the preorthosis fracture rate.[10, 40] An intensive study is presently underway at NIH-CHNMC to evaluate the effects of aggressive rehabilitation, including orthotic use, on ambulation, bone density, and disease morbidity in children with osteogenesis imperfecta.

Reciprocating Gait Orthoses (Fig. 9–10)

Several studies have compared the energy efficiency of ambulation with RGOs compared to HKAFOs for children with myelomeningocele. With RGOs, ambulation velocity was found to increase, whereas energy expenditure, as evidenced by pulse rate, decreased.[41, 42, 66] McCall and Schmidt[42] studied 41 children with myelomeningocele ambulating under three condi-

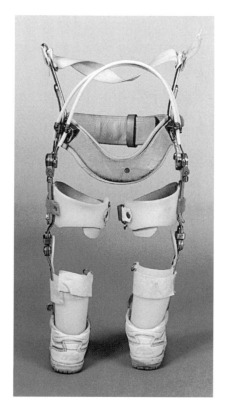

FIGURE 9–10. Reciprocating gait orthosis (RGO) with thoracic strap, posterior view.

tions: wearing RGOs with the cable released, which allowed full hip flexion; wearing RGOs with hips and knees locked to simulate a swing-through gait; and wearing HKAFOs and RGOs in the standard configuration. The children ambulated 30 feet at their maximum speed under the three bracing conditions while velocity and pulse rate were recorded. McCall and Schmidt[42] reported lower pulse rates and higher walking velocities for 31 of the children wearing the RGOs in the standard configuration. However, a significant difference between ambulation with standard RGOs and RGOs with locked hips and knees was not reported. A 3-year follow-up report on the children by McCall showed that 78% of the children achieved the level of household or community ambulation using the RGOs in the standard configuration. In an earlier study, Hoffer and colleagues[28] reported that of 56 children with myelomeningocele who used HKAFOs and a swing-through pattern for ambulation, only 35% achieved a level of household or community ambulation.

ORTHOSES FOR CHILDREN WITH NEUROLOGIC INVOLVEMENT

Chapter 8 reviews normal gait and the consequences of neurologic abnormalities on a functional gait pattern. In similarity with the gait of adults with neurologic involvement, the gait of children with cerebral palsy is characterized by insufficient generation of force, abnormal electromyographic activity, and decreased moment of force output of affected muscle groups.[7, 47] Functionally, these abnormalities may be manifested as decreased walking velocity, decreased stride length, and increased energy cost when compared to normal children of comparable ages.[46, 47] Clinically, the child may present with abnormal stance postures, range-of-motion limitations, and delayed or inappropriate balance responses.

In the treatment of cerebral palsy over the years, orthoses have either been used with enthusiasm or have been replaced by alternative treatments. For children with cerebral palsy, orthoses have generally been used to prevent or reduce contractures, to prevent secondary impairment, and to promote function. Orthoses aid some children if the purpose of the device is well defined. Conversely, they may be harmless, but not beneficial, to other children, and they have the potential to produce secondary deformities or impairments when the goal is not clearly defined and their use is not closely monitored.

Various types of orthoses have been used to improve or prevent range-of-motion limitations and to prevent secondary deformities such as hip dislocations and torsional problems.[12] Few studies address the effectiveness of orthoses in the prevention of secondary limitations. Baumann and Zumstein[4] recommend the use of the clamshell type ankle-foot orthosis (AFO) during sleep as a method to prevent ankle plantarflexion contractures. In this study, yearly recordings were made of the passive range of motion of the ankles, knees, and hips of children with cerebral palsy from 3 years of age through the end of the skeletal growth period. The children wore the clamshell AFO at night throughout this time period. The results indicated that long-term prevention of plantarflexion contractures with surgery for an equinous foot deformity was very rare for the children in this study. The sample size of 1200 orthoses for this study was large, but the actual numbers of children requiring surgery were not discussed. A disadvantage of this method of management is the length of time that the orthosis is required to be worn and the obvious difficulties of compliance, possible skin breakdown, and cost. In his experience, Bleck[12] found that HKAFOs did not prevent hip flexion contractures or hip dislocations. Medical professionals must clearly define the goals to be achieved with the orthosis and monitor the effectiveness of the orthosis if maximum benefits are to be realized.

In the 1980s, several studies addressed the use of inhibitive casts on the ability to improve gait parameters of stride and step length, base of support, and heel contact. Inhibitive casts are short plaster or fiberglass leg casts that incorporate a foot plate with areas of relief to decrease the influence of tonic foot reflexes. Bertoti[9] and Hinderer and colleagues[27] reported significant improvements in stride length for children treated with inhibitive casts compared to children receiving other treatment. Bertoti studied eight children and a control group for a 10-week period with casts, whereas Hinderer and colleagues reported on two children and used a single-subject design with repeated measures. Neither study assessed the long-term carry-over effects of wearing the cast. Watt et al[64] demonstrated improvements in passive ankle dorsiflexion and foot contact during gait in a study of 28 children with cerebral palsy treated with inhibitive casts. The improvements in passive ankle dorsiflexion range of motion were maintained for 2 weeks after the cast was applied, but the ankle dorsiflexion range of motion had returned to baseline values when measured 5 months postapplication. Short leg casts or inhibitive casts are messy to apply, time-consuming to fabricate, and cumbersome for the user. For clinical use, they have been replaced by both high- and low-temperature thermoplastic AFOs.

More recently, Mossberg and colleagues[45] examined the effects of orthoses on functional outcome in children with cerebral palsy. Energy expenditure was evaluated in children with spastic diplegia walking at self-selected speeds with and without their prescribed AFOs. The investigators reported that the children expended less energy when ambulating with the AFOs compared to ambulating without the AFOs; the differences, however, were not statistically significant.

Many children with spastic diplegia may ambulate with hinged AFOs instead of with solid AFOs. The purpose of a hinged AFO is to allow ankle dorsiflexion with knee flexion at midstance so that the tibia may advance forward over the foot in preparation for terminal stance. In a kinematic case study of a child with spastic diplegia, Middleton and associates[43] compared the use of hinged AFOs and solid AFOs during gait. With the child wearing the hinged AFO, the ankle dorsiflexion pattern during stance resembled a more normal pattern. Baker and colleagues[3] compared the hinged AFOs and fixed (solid) AFOs during a sit-to-stand task in ten children with cerebral palsy. The investigators found statistically significant increases in trunk lean angles during rising from the sit-to-stand position when the children wore the fixed AFOs compared to the hinged AFOs. These authors suggest that the type of AFO may influence movement strategies when functional tasks are being performed. A study by Knutson[36] compared the use of no orthosis, fixed AFOs, or hinged AFOs on kinematic and electromyographic changes in 15 children with cerebral palsy. Ambulation velocity was increased in children wearing the hinged AFOs, and ankle dorsiflexion at midstance of gait was increased. These initial studies suggest that the use of hinged AFOs may lead to functional improvements in gait for children with cerebral palsy or spastic diplegia.

Inhibitive AFOs combine the use of the polypropylene materials used in the fabrication of AFOs with the "inhibitive" aspects of casting, and several authors have reported on the treatment of children with cerebral palsy with inhibitive AFOs. Using a single-subject alternating-treatment design, Harris and Riffle[23] evaluated the effects of an inhibitive AFO on the standing balance of a child with cerebral palsy. A longer duration of independent standing was obtained when the child wore the inhibitive AFO. Taylor and Harris[61] presented a case study that evaluated the effects of an inhibitive AFO on the functional motor performance of a child with cerebral palsy. The child was assessed with and without inhibitive AFOs for standing balance, ball-catching activities, and score on the fine-motor portion of the Peabody Developmental Motor Scale. No quantitative differences were obtained with standing balance or ball catching with or without the inhibitive AFOs. The child's performance on the Peabody fine-motor scale was at age level for two out of three areas when the inhibitive AFOs were worn and below one standard deviation from the mean in all three fine-motor areas when the inhibitive AFOs were not worn. Neither group of investigators clearly defined the term "inhibitive AFO." Because the use of AFOs is advocated for improvements in gait and stance, further studies are needed in these areas to document their efficacy in children with cerebral palsy.

Ricks and Eilert[53] evaluated the effects of inhibitory casts and orthoses on maintaining bone alignment during weight bearing with inhibitive casts, inhibitive AFOs, inhibitive articulating AFOs, or bare feet. The investigators found that bone alignment was not maintained during weight bearing with the various inhibitive orthoses. They proposed that orthotic devices could be constructed to inhibit spasticity and speculated that "pressure concentrated over certain bones might inhibit reflexes or abnormal muscle tone in the foot," which may produce improvements in the child's balance or gait.

The literature also contains reports of the use of dynamic AFOs (DAFOs)

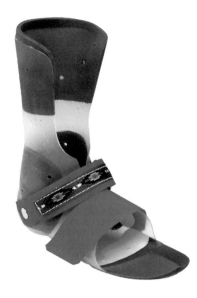

FIGURE 9–11. DAFO #3, Plantarflexion block. (Courtesy of Cascade Prosthetics and Orthotics Inc., Bellingham, Washington.)

in children with cerebral palsy. Hylton[30] defines a DAFO as a thin flexible supramalleolar orthosis with a custom-contoured soleplate (footboard) to provide support and stabilize the dynamic arches of the foot. (Fig. 9–11). DAFOs allow varying degrees of ankle plantarflexion and dorsiflexion while providing mediolateral control. Hylton proposed that DAFOs have three beneficial effects: (1) the total contact fit is more easily tolerated and skin breakdown problems are negligible; (2) the stability and proprioceptive feedback provided by a DAFO assists the user with balance and postural control; and (3) the custom-contoured footboard provides support to the natural arch contours of the foot. Hylton advocates the use of DAFOs in conjunction with active postural control and a balance-oriented therapy program, and supports the need for research to document the effectiveness of DAFOs for children with neurologic involvement. Subjective clinical findings reported by Hylton[30] include ease of positioning in wheelchairs and standers and improvements in oral motor control, postural and tone control, standing balance, weight bearing for a child with hemiplegia, and use of the involved arm for a child with hemiplegia. Bailes and Donohoe-Follmore[2] compared the effect of an articulated AFO, a supramalleolar DAFO, or bare feet on the standing balance of a child recovering from a head injury. The standing balance was longer when the child wore the DAFO, and clinically, the standing balance reactions were more appropriate when the child was wearing the DAFO.

Cascade Prosthetics and Orthotics[14] (Bellingham, WA) fabricates various styles of DAFOs (Fig. 9–12). According to Cascade Prosthetics and Orthotics, the purpose of the DAFO is to provide midline stability and control or inhibition of abnormal hypertonus in the lower extremities. The various

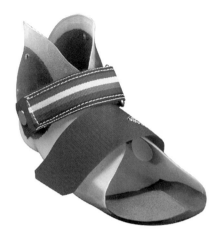

FIGURE 9–12. DAFO #4, Plantarflexion free. (Courtesy of Cascade Prosthetics and Orthotics Inc., Bellingham, Washington.)

styles of orthoses aim to correct different alignment problems and to promote functions appropriate for the particular child using the orthosis.

A review of the literature reveals the confusion concerning orthosis use for children with neurologic involvement. The factors contributing to this confusion include the following: a variety of names exist for very similar orthoses; well-defined studies to validate the use of various orthoses are lacking; and unsubstantiated claims are made of distal control of abnormal neurologic responses that effect changes throughout a limb or even within the central nervous system itself.

Two questions that the clinician treating the child with neurologic involvement must address before prescribing an orthosis are Which orthotic device will benefit the child? and What are those benefits? Harris'[24] criteria for evaluating the scientific merit of a treatment approach may assist the clinician in reaching a decision. The six criteria that should be met before a treatment or new technique is prescribed are the following: (1) valid anatomic and physiologic evidence exists to support the treatment approach; (2) the treatment approach is designed for a specific population; (3) potential side effects of the treatment approach are presented; (4) peer-reviewed journals support the treatment efficacy; (5) peer-reviewed studies exist; and (6) proponents of the treatment approach discuss its limitations.

Many of the orthoses currently in use for children with neurologic involvement do not meet these criteria. Health-care providers do not need to abandon the use of these devices, but they do need to substantiate their use and limit the claims of their effectiveness until proof is obtained. Studies in the literature are beginning to delineate the uses of hinged and solid AFOs for specific populations and for improvement of certain motor tasks. More studies are needed in this area. For example, two separate well-defined studies have examined the effects of inhibitive AFOs on standing balance, but the results were not in agreement, substantiating the need for further investigation.[23, 61]

Several of the previously discussed studies attempted to explain the improvements or lack of improvements according to physiologic principles. This is an important step for acceptance by the scientific community, but the anatomic or physiologic principles proposed need to be verified and substantiated in the literature.

In conclusion, many of the orthoses discussed for children with various *orthopedic* diagnoses meet Harris' six criteria. New orthoses to limit negative side effects and improve outcomes still need to be developed. Health-care providers should bear the responsibility for evaluating the theoretical basis and effectiveness of the newer orthoses, as well as of those currently available for children with neurologic involvement, before fully endorsing their use and making claims to patients, their families, and third-party payers. Thus, the children who are served will be ensured safe and effective methods of treatment.

REFERENCES

1. Arkin AM, Katz JF: The effects of pressure on epiphyseal growth. J Bone Joint Surg 38A:1056–1076, 1956.
2. Bailes AF, Donohoe-Follmore B: Comparison of articulating AFOB and dynamic AFOB used with a child during recovery from a head injury—a case study. Pediatr Phys Ther 7:199, 1995.
3. Baker MJ, Giuliani CA, Sparling J, Schenkman ML: Effects of ankle-foot orthosis on a sit-to-stand task in children with cerebral palsy. Pediatr Phys Ther 5:193, 1993.
4. Baumann JM, Zumstein M: Experience with a plastic ankle-foot orthosis for prevention of muscle contracture. Dev Med Child Neurol 27:83, 1985.
5. Beals RK: Developmental changes in the femur and acetabulum in spastic paraplegia and diplegia. Dev Med Child Neurol 11:303–313, 1969.
6. Beaty JH: Developmental Problems in the Lower Extremity. In Canale ST, Beaty JH (eds): Operative Pediatric Orthopedics. St. Louis, Mosby-Year Book, 1991, pp 357–370.
7. Berger W, Quintern J, Deitz V: Pathophysiology of gait in children with cerebral palsy. Electroencephalogr Clin Neurophysiol 53:538–548, 1992.
8. Bernhardt DB: Prenatal and postnatal growth and development of the foot and ankle. Phys Ther 68:1831–1839, 1988.
9. Bertoti DB: Effects of short leg casting on ambulation in children with cerebral palsy. Phys Ther 66:1522–1529, 1986.
10. Binder H, Hawks L, Graybull G, et al: Osteogenesis imperfecta: rehabilitation approach with infants and young children. Arch Phys Med Rehab 65:537–541, 1984.
11. Bleck EE: Developmental orthopedics III: toddlers. Dev Med Child Neurol 24:533–555, 1982.
12. Bleck EE: Orthopedic Management in Cerebral Palsy. Philadelphia, J.B. Lippincott, 1987.
13. Canale ST: Osteochondroses. In Canale ST, Beaty JH (eds): Operative Pediatric Orthopedics. St. Louis, Mosby-Year Book, 1991, pp 743–776.
14. Cascade Prosthetics and Orthotics: Cascade Dynamic Ankle Foot Orthotics. Bellingham, WA, Cascade Prosthetics and Orthotics, 1996
15. Catterall A: The natural history of perthes disease. J Bone Joint Surg 53B:37–53, 1971.
16. Cunningham E, McCulloch P, Schenkman M: The evaluation of weight bearing in children with cerebral palsy on prone, supine, and upright standers. Pediatr Phys Ther 4:193, 1992.
17. Curtis BH, Gunther SF, Gossling HR, et al: Treatment for Legg-Perthes disease with the Newington abduction brace. J Bone Joint Surg 56A:1135–1146, 1974.

18. Cusick BD, Stuberg WA: Assessment of lower-extremity alignment in the transverse plane: implications for management of children with neuromotor dysfunction. Phys Ther 72:3–15, 1992.
19. Denton JR: Experience with Legg-Calvé-Perthes disease 1968–1974 at the New York Orthopedic Hospital. Clin Orthop 150:36–41, 1980.
20. Drennan JC: Orthotic management of the myelomeningocele spine. Dev Med Child Neurol 18 (suppl 37):935–946, 1976.
22. Dunne KB, Clarren SK: The origin of prenatal and postnatal deformities. Pediatr Clin North Am 33:1277–1297, 1986.
23. Harris SR, Riffle K: Effects of inhibitive ankle-foot orthoses on standing balance in a child with cerebral palsy. Phys Ther 66:663–667, 1986.
24. Harris SR: How should treatments be critiqued for scientific merit? Phys Ther 76:175–181, 1996.
25. Heikkila E: Comparison of the Frejka pillow and von Rosen splint in treatment of congenital dislocation of the hip. J Pediatr Orthop 8:20–24, 1988.
26. Hensinger RN: Congenital dislocation of the hip, treatment in infancy to walking age. Orthop Clin North Am 18:597–616, 1987.
27. Hinderer KA, Harris SR, Purdy AH, et al: Effects of "tone-reducing" casts vs. standard plaster-cast on gait improvement of children with cerebral palsy. Dev Med Child Neurol 30:370–377, 1988.
28. Hoffer M, Feiwell E, Perry R, et al: Functional ambulation in patients with myelomeningocele. J Bone Joint Surg Am 55:137–148, 1973.
29. Howard CB, McKibbon B, Williams LA: Factors affecting the incidence of hip dislocation in cerebral palsy. J Bone Joint Surg 67:530–532, 1985.
30. Hylton NM: Postural and functional impact of dynamic AFO's and FO's in a pediatric population. J Prosthet Orthot 2:40–53, 1989.
31. Jeffries LM, McEwen IR, Venkataram PS, et al: Relations among age, weight, bone mineral content, and bone mineral density in children with spastic cerebral palsy and children without disabilities. Pediatr Phys Ther 6:210, 1994.
32. Kalamchi A, MacFarlane R: The pavlik harness: results in patients over three months of age. J Pediatr Orthop 2:3–8, 1982.
33. Katz JF: Legg-Calve-Perthes disease: results of treatment. Clin Orthop 10:61–78, 1957.
34. Knittel G, Staheli LT: The effectiveness of shoe modifications for intoeing. Orthop Clin North Am 7:1019–1025, 1976.
35. Knutson LM, Clark DE: Orthotic devices for ambulation in children with cerebral palsy and myelomeningocele. Phys Ther 71:947–960, 1991.
36. Knutson LM: The effects of fixed and hinged ankle foot orthoses on gait myoelectric activity and standing joint alignment in children with cerebral palsy. Unpublished dissertation, University of Iowa, Iowa City, IA, 1993.
37. LeVeau BF, Bernhardt DB: Developmental biomechanics: effects of forces on the growth, development, and maintenance of the human body. Phys Ther 64:1874–1882, 1984.
38. Lock TR, Aronson DD: Fractures in patients with myelomeningocele. J Bone Joint Surg 71A:1153–1157, 1989.
39. Lough LK, Nielson DH: Ambulation of children with myelomeningocele: parapodium versus parapodium with Orlau swivel modification. Dev Med Child Neurol 28:489–497, 1986.
40. Marini JC: Osteogenesis imperfecta: comprehensive management. In Barness LA (Eds): Advances in Pediatrics. St. Louis, Mosby-Year Book, 1988, pp 391–426.
41. Mazur JM, Shurtleff D, Menelaus M, et al: Orthopedic management of high-level spina bifida. J Bone Joint Surg 71A:56–61, 1989.
42. McCall RE, Schmidt WT: Clinical experiences with the reciprocal gait orthosis in myelodysplasia. J Pediatr Orthop 6:157–161, 1986.
43. Middleton EA, Hurley GRB, McIlwain JS: The role of rigid and hinged polypropylene ankle-foot-orthosis in the management of cerebral palsy: a case study. Prosthet Orthot Int 12:129–135, 1988.
44. Miedaner J: An evaluation of weight bearing forces at various standing angles for children with cerebral palsy. Pediatr Phys Ther 2:215, 1990.
45. Mossberg KA, Linton KA, Friske K: Ankle-foot orthoses: effect on energy expenditure of gait in spastic diplegic children. Arch Phys Med Rehab 71:490–494, 1990.
46. Norlin R, Odenrick P: Development of gait in spastic children with cerebral palsy. J Pediatr Orthoped 6:674–680, 1986.

47. Olney SJ, Wright MJ: Cerebral palsy. In Campbell SK (Ed): Physical Therapy for Children. Philadelphia, W.B. Saunders Co., 1994, pp 489–524.
48. Pavlik A: The functional method of treatment using a harness with stirrups as the primary method of conservative therapy for infants with congenital dislocation of the hip. Clin Orthop 281:4–10, 1992.
49. Petrie JB, Bitnec I: The abduction weight-bearing treatment in Legg-Perthes disease. J Bone Joint Surg 53B:54, 1971.
50. Phelps WM: Prevention of acquired dislocation of the hip in cerebral palsy. J Bone Joint Surg Am 41:440–448, 1959.
51. Purvis JM, Dimon JH, Meehan PL, et al: Preliminary experience with the Scottish Rite Hospital abduction orthosis for Legg-Perthes disease. Clin Orthop 150:49–53, 1980.
52. Ralis ZA, Ralis HM, Randall M, et al: Changes in shape, ossification and quality of bones in children with spina bifida. Dev Med Child Neurol 18 (suppl 37):29–41, 1976.
53. Ricks NR, Eilert RE: Effects of inhibitory casts and orthoses on bony alignment of foot and ankle during weight-bearing in children with spasticity. Dev Med Child Neurol 35:11–16, 1993.
54. Rosenstein BD, Greene WB, Herrington RT, et al: Bone density in myelomeningocele: the effects of ambulatory status and other factors. Dev Med Child Neurol 29:486–494, 1987.
55. Ryan KD, Ploski C, Emans JB: Myelodysplasia—the musculoskeletal problem: habilitation from infancy to adulthood. Phys Ther 71:935–946, 1991.
56. Staheli LT: Torsional deformity. Pediatr Clin North Am 24:799–811, 1977.
57. Staheli LT, Corbett M, Wyss C, et al: Lower-extremity rotational problems in children. J Bone Joint Surg 67A:39–47, 1985.
58. Staheli LT: Torsion-treatment indications. Clin Orthop 247:61–66, 1989.
59. Stuberg WA: Considerations related to weight-bearing programs in children with developmental disabilities. Phys Ther 72:35–40, 1992.
60. Tachdjian MO: Pediatric Orthopedics, 2nd ed., Vol 1–4. Philadelphia, W.B. Saunders Co., 1990.
61. Taylor CL, Harris SR: Effects of ankle-foot orthoses on functional motor performance in a child with spastic diplegia. Am J Occup Ther 40:492–494, 1986.
62. Thompson GH, Salter RB: Legg-Calve-Perthes disease. Orthop Clin North Am 18:617–635, 1987.
63. Walker JM: Musculoskeletal development: a review. Phys Ther 71:878–889, 1991.
64. Watt J, Sims D, Harckham F, et al: A prospective study of inhibitive casting as an adjunct to physiotherapy for cerebral-palsied children. Dev Med Child Neurol 28:480–488, 1986.
65. Wenger DR, Ward WT, Herring JA: Current concepts review Legg-Calvé-Perthes disease. J Bone Joint Surg 73A:778–788, 1991.
66. Yngve DA, Douglas R, Roberts JM: The reciprocating gait orthosis in myelomeningocele. J Pediatr Orthop 4:304–310, 1984.

Index